MW01178862

Towards Individualized Therapy for Multiple Myeloma

A Guide for Choosing Treatment that Best Fits Patients

Towards Individualized Therapy for Multiple Myeloma

A Guide for Choosing Treatment that Best Fits Patients

Gerrard Teoh

Gleneagles Hospital, Singapore

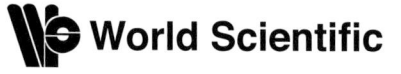 **World Scientific**

NEW JERSEY · LONDON · SINGAPORE · BEIJING · SHANGHAI · HONG KONG · TAIPEI · CHENNAI

Published by

World Scientific Publishing Co. Pte. Ltd.

5 Toh Tuck Link, Singapore 596224

USA office: 27 Warren Street, Suite 401-402, Hackensack, NJ 07601

UK office: 57 Shelton Street, Covent Garden, London WC2H 9HE

British Library Cataloguing-in-Publication Data
A catalogue record for this book is available from the British Library.

TOWARDS INDIVIDUALIZED THERAPY FOR MULTIPLE MYELOMA
A Guide for Choosing Treatment that Best Fits Patients

Copyright © 2009 by World Scientific Publishing Co. Pte. Ltd.

All rights reserved. This book, or parts thereof, may not be reproduced in any form or by any means, electronic or mechanical, including photocopying, recording or any information storage and retrieval system now known or to be invented, without written permission from the Publisher.

For photocopying of material in this volume, please pay a copying fee through the Copyright Clearance Center, Inc., 222 Rosewood Drive, Danvers, MA 01923, USA. In this case permission to photocopy is not required from the publisher.

ISBN-13 978-981-283-579-6 (pbk)
ISBN-10 981-283-579-2 (pbk)

Typeset by Stallion Press
Email: enquiries@stallionpress.com

Printed by FuIsland Offset Printing (S) Pte Ltd, Singapore

To Alice, Gaius and Abital, with Love;
and
Ken for Believing in Me

PROLOGUE

"I believe that patients will do better with their treatment when their doctors communicate information more effectively to them."

Ever so often I meet a patient who looks me in the eye and smiles inappropriately and almost mockingly, who then suggests that I should rephrase myself so that I could be better understood. Whilst this is certainly not an unfamiliar situation for many doctors, I will not make excuses for our breed for our inability to communicate with the layperson. Let's admit it guys, we doctors are often so easily carried away by the science and jargon of our world that we unconsciously leave our poor patients behind at the starting blocks to figure things out on their own. We don't seem to realize that when we communicate information that is difficult to comprehend, patients are forced by our insensitivities to come to their own conclusions about their health. You cannot blame your patients if they come to a flawed conclusion or one with a wild twist. But fortunately for us, most of our patients ultimately find the correct answers. The problem is we doctors are not living in the real world. Many of us literally don't even see the lights of day. To make things worse, medical science has of late become frenetic in churning out new knowledge. There's barely enough time for the dust to settle before more data comes in. I am thoroughly convinced that it is frankly impossible for the layman to figure things

vii

out. Despite all that's on the internet; or more precisely because of all that's (misleading) on the internet, laypeople shouldn't even try. There are less painful ways of doing this. I know all patients want to have everything and have it in a logical package. But manage your expectations, the logic is at best 80%, the rest of the 20% is still chaos. This book will hopefully give you enough of the groundwork to start some logical reasoning. If you can't even understand this book, take heart that you're normal and get on with the more important issues of getting well.

This book is deliberately written in everyday English and in a lighter mood for the benefit of those of us who visit doctors but don't really understand what the doctor said. It is meant primarily for patients with multiple myeloma[a] (MM). However, this book may also be a valuable resource for family members, friends, doctors, nurses, as well as anyone else who is interested in considering a more-than-worthy alternative mode of therapy for MM, i.e. other than standard therapy. The author has the opinion that what has been loosely termed as "standard therapy" is (frequently) not necessarily the best form of treatment at all for patients with MM. In his experience, patients come in all shapes and sizes, so having only one size of whatever therapy will certainly not work for every patient.

Serendipitously, MM patients are spoilt for choice today. Exponential increases in bench-to-bedside (translational[b]) research spending by academic and commercial agencies have greatly: (i) increased our current understanding of MM biology, (ii) accelerated the pace

---

[a] My mentor in Harvard Medical School, Prof Kenneth Anderson, considered MM to be totally evil, and would not tolerate capitalization of the term "multiple myeloma" when written; as that would give the disease more respect that necessary. Ken was often right...

[b] Basic Research refers to very fundamental studies performed usually in a laboratory. When the results of such research (e.g. a molecule) is used (or applied) to create a product (e.g. a drug) that can be used for clinical treatment, this is often called Applied Research. The final step of bringing this product from the research bench to the patient requires rigorous testing in the laboratory (*in vitro* testing), perhaps in research animals (*in vivo* testing), and finally in human clinical trials. This complex process is also called Translational Research.

Prologue ix

of novel drug discovery, (iii) improved therapeutic drug targeting, and (iv) expanded patient access to these novel therapies. In other words, patients now have the luxury of picking and choosing from not just a few, but numerous new "designer" therapeutic compounds that have recently flooded the market. Accordingly, patients (and their doctors) can tailor their treatments to suit their diseases, their lifestyles, and most importantly, their pockets. Without a doubt, "boutique" medicines are the IN things for patients with MM. Costs aside, patients are no more bothered by treatments that might not work; today, they can "swatch" (mix and match) confidently between different highly-effective compounds to achieve: (i) better disease control, (ii) better adverse effects profiles, and (iii) more holistic healthcare programs that potentially result in "cure".

The key to better therapeutic outcomes via individualizing of anti-MM therapy is an in-depth understanding of the group dynamics that dictate the algorithms surrounding the way doctors decide therapy. This is a no-brainer; things do not happen alone, they always affect the group. Enhancing or suppressing an aspect of treatment and/or response to treatment will lead to group effects within that single individual. It is vital to separate this concept from what the author considers as the most confounding information that can be gleaned (especially from the internet) by patients. It is what we know of, and unfortunately strive for in healthcare accreditation exercises, as evidence-based medicine (EBM) i.e. the artificial world of clinical trials.

Patients undergoing clinical trials are a highly-selected group of individuals who are required to fulfill stringent eligibility criteria. They are then subjected to fixed treatment regimens that have been designed by groups of investigators (usually renowned doctors) and representatives from the pharmaceutical (sponsoring) companies. Because of tight controls during the conduct of these trials, including strict rules that govern how data should be collected, one size is made to fit all, or else patients simply fall-out of the study. The data so obtained, with all these and more biases built in, is now deemed as medical "evidence". When in actual fact what it is, is nothing really more than a statistical valuation of that regimen in a highly confined cohort of patients.

Unfortunately, this information is then marketed as "truth" (for want of a better word), and frequently extrapolated to all patients, regardless of shape and/or size. Sadly, the actual physicians who advocate EBM might in fact be the most ill-informed lot; believing that they are doing their best at convincing patients to undertake certain therapies that could well be totally inapplicable. The author does not in any way discount the value of doing good clinical studies. He is in fact the principal investigator of a number of clinical trials. The author is only cautioning against the random extrapolation of such information, and the potential "accidental" misinformation that could occur when these study results are quoted to patients, who are by-and-large ignorant of the clinical trials processes. This fundamental point cannot be over-stated. Ultimately, a patient's treatment is a very personal thing, and it has to be individualized, regardless of the clinical evidence. As a patient, the best treatment for you is simply the one that works, regardless of formal clinical evidence. And vice versa, the worst treatment you can receive will be the one that is thought to work for you but in reality does not fit you at all. You are you, an individual, and to you treatment must be individualized to suit you first.

CONTENTS

Prologue		vii
Chapter 1.	Introduction	1
Chapter 2.	Diagnostic Dilemmas	8
Chapter 3.	Shortcomings of Modern-Day Clinical Trials	20
Chapter 4.	Individualizing Core Parameters	28
Chapter 5.	Patient Compliance	49
Chapter 6.	Multiple Myeloma	72
Chapter 7.	Current Treatment	140
Chapter 8.	Future Opportunities	150
Chapter 9.	Concluding Remarks	157
Abbreviations		159
Glossary		163
List of Figures		173
List of Tables		177
References		179
Index		187

Chapter **1**

INTRODUCTION

"3 Cases of MM"

If you already know what MM is, you might still want to read on because I will be discussing an interesting dilemma that we as hematologists face today when treating patients with MM. If you don't know what MM is, you obviously must read on so that you will understand your doctors a little better when you next meet them. Multiple myeloma is a blood or hematological cancer. In Latin, "myelo" means bone marrow (BM), and "oma" means tumor or cancer. Hence, "myeloma" is a bone marrow cancer. In our bodies, the BM is found inside our bones. As you know, our skeleton is made up of many bones but not all the bones contain marrow. By and large, BM is found inside the larger bones. Moreover, when we are younger, more of the skeleton contains active marrow; but as we age, some of the BM "dries up," as it were, and some of the bones that originally contained marrow now become devoid of it. Multiple myeloma is called "multiple" because it is often found in many separate sites in the BM of our skeleton at the time of diagnosis. The cancerous myeloma cell is a malignant plasma cell. The normal counterparts of this cell, i.e. normal plasma cells, are cells of the immune system that produce antibodies (Ab), also known as immunoglobulins (Ig), in our bodies. Antibodies protect us from invasion by foreign agents, e.g. germs. One plasma cell (of the immune system) will produce only one type of Ab. This is the concept of monoclonality. However, during an infection,

1

e.g. influenza, many plasma cells are activated and together they produce numerous different types of Igs that fight the flu virus. Such a concerted Ab response by many normal plasma cells is also called a polyclonal Ab response.

The situation is different in MM where only one plasma cell had at the outset become cancerous. Over time this cancerous cell multiplied itself through numerous cell divisions and gave rise to many copies or clones of itself. Each member of this clone of malignant plasma cells produces the same Ab or Ig (e.g. Ig class G or IgG). Ultimately, the Abs that are secreted by this clone of MM cells are identical and are called monoclonal Abs (mAbs). In the context of MM, these mAbs are also called monoclonal proteins or myeloma proteins or M-proteins. Because MM cells arise in the BM, normal blood production and blood counts may be affected by the presence of the cancer, i.e. suppressed (e.g. patients may have anemia). Hence, in established MM, patients often complain of fatigue and poor immunity. Moreover, because the BM is found inside the bones of the skeleton, patients with MM also frequently complain of bone pain and high blood calcium levels (hypercalcemia) because of bone destruction, i.e. MM bone disease. Furthermore, because the smaller component parts of the Ig molecule (also called the light chains) are able to pass through the filtering system of the kidneys (the glomeruli), and are capable of inducing toxic reactions in the tubes of the kidneys (the renal tubules), M-protein light chains can lead to varying degrees of kidney (renal) failure. In summary, hypercalcemia, renal failure, anemia and bone pain/disease, which form the acronym "CRAB," are the clinical hallmarks of MM. In the presence of at least some of the clinical features outlined by "CRAB," the diagnosis of MM is confirmed by the biochemical identification of the M-protein and the presence of malignant plasma cells in the BM sample.

Case 1. A Typical MM Patient

At about 3:00 p.m. on a hot and humid afternoon, a 45-year-old lorry driver was having a late lunch at work when he suddenly lost his balance and fell from his chair and onto the floor, hitting his head on the floor in the process. He had apparently fractured his right hip and was writhing in pain, almost to the point of delirium. The cause of the injury was trivial — he had reached forward and towards his right to pick up his newspapers to read when the upper part of his right leg snapped into two. This was quite evident on the X-rays that were subsequently taken at the Accident and Emergency department.

Further X-rays demonstrated multiple small spherical lesions in the hip and leg bones, as well as in the skull, that resembled bones that had been moth-eaten. These multiple bone tumors, called lytic lesions,[c] were typical findings of MM bone disease. Indeed, the whole skeleton could be riddled by these lytic lesions, thus making the bones very brittle. At the slightest injury, these bones could simply fracture — so-called pathological fractures. Because the fracture site does not contain bone or bone cells, but rather cancer cells, bone healing is frequently slow or impossible, and bone pain intractable. Indeed, MM is one of the most painful cancers that we know of. Through other laboratory tests, it was subsequently found that this patient had hypercalcemia, anemia and renal impairment, all the hallmarks of MM. Biochemical tests also confirmed the presence of the M-protein, which was of the subtype IgGκ[d] (for immunoglobulin G and the kappa light chain (LC) subtype). He went on to receive standard therapy for MM and died two-and-a-half years later.

Case 2. A Less Obvious Case of MM

A frail 94-year-old woman was being nursed in the Medical Intensive Care Unit (ICU) of a local hospital. She was a domestic helper in

---

[c] In Latin, the term for bone is "osteo-". Thinning of bone is also known as osteopenia. When bone thinning is marked in a certain area, that lesion is called an osteolytic lesion. By contrast, in some diseases bone formation is increased in certain areas. This kind of lesion is called an osteoblastic lesion.

[d] The common subtypes of MM are IgG and IgA; with either kappa or lambda light chains. For example IgGκ, IgGλ, IgAκ or IgAλ.

her youth, and a relatively petit and quiet woman who rarely complained about any sickness. A fall whilst walking in the rain a fortnight ago had changed her life completely. She had been unconscious ever since. A hairline fracture at the back of her skull and multiple broken ribs were detected by X-rays. After three days in hospital, she developed a fearsome fever due to widespread pneumonia in both lungs. Despite the use of antibiotics, her condition continued to deteriorate and decompensate.

She was nursed in the Medical ICU because of a dangerously low blood pressure, so low that augmentation using continuous intravenous medication (called inotropes) had to be instituted. Moreover, she required repeated blood transfusions for persistent anemia. Serial chest X-rays performed to monitor her pneumonia revealed that some of the rib fractures were actually old fractures that had most likely preceded her fall by a number of months. To the trained eye, some degree of bone healing had already taken place in these fractures. In other words, she already had rib fractures that she didn't even know of, again typical of pathological fractures. A very mild hypercalcemia and mild renal impairment alerted her doctors to the possibility that she could have MM. The appropriate investigations were performed and these confirmed that she indeed had an IgGκ MM.

Because she was very sick, it was decided that treatment would be attenuated (individualized). An extremely gentle regimen comprising 5 mg of prednisolone (Pred, a steroid or glucocorticoid) once a day was selected for her MM. After just four days of therapy, her fever settled and she regained consciousness. After another two weeks of treatment, she was discharged from hospital and returned home in a wheelchair. This patient continued to be given higher daily doses of Pred for several more months but she finally succumbed to her MM. Her treatment was individualized and palliative (i.e. not curative and not for prolonging survival), the aim being to give her the best quality of life (QoL) possible.

Introduction 5

Case 3. Does this Patient have MM?

The next patient is one of the most difficult MM cases that I have ever diagnosed. I wonder till today if the delay in diagnosis has had made a difference to the outcome of his treatment. This is a 60-year-old man, who has worked for many years as a welder before he was admitted to a local hospital for severe backache. Apparently, he was otherwise a relatively fit chap, and was watching television when he developed an acute and severe backache. He described himself as being hit in the lower back by a torpedo and had become immediately incapacitated by excruciating pain. He couldn't even turn about in bed or bathe himself.

As expected, he was admitted under the Orthopedic Service, and underwent magnetic resonance imaging (MRI) scanning within hours of admission. The MRI scan was completely normal. Moreover, a radionuclide bone scan was also negative and no further orthopedic intervention was performed. He was then transferred to the Neurology Service for further testing. A whole barrage of tests was done, including lumbar puncture (LP), but all these tests were again negative. Pain continued to be severe and was relieved only by high doses of opiate-based medicines like morphine. As a result, he developed severe nausea and vomiting, ileus (paralysis of the gut) and constipation and was referred to the Gastroenterology Service. Yet again, further tests were carried out, including computerized tomographic (CT) scans, gastroscopy and colonoscopy. Again no abnormalities of the abdominal organs were detected. It was not difficult to understand his frustration.

"My pain is so bad," he said, "I cannot sleep. I take so much morphine; I'm worried I will be addicted. So I ask for sleeping pills. But the doctors say I can also be addicted to sleeping pills and cannot take too many of those. I vomit or cannot pass motion every time I take morphine. I really feel like dying."

All his routine blood and urine tests were normal except for borderline hypercalcemia and increased Igs. He was then suspected to have MM and I was called to review him. Unfortunately, all the specific MM studies, BM studies and full skeletal survey were also negative. The Ig fraction was in fact polyclonal[e] and a good healthy BM was found when examined. To all intents and purposes, MM could be ruled out. But my suspicions of MM continued to be high, and I then asked for a bone mineral density (BMD) dual-energy X-ray absorptiometry (DXA or DEXA) scan to be done. This showed severe osteopenia with bone thinning well below three standard deviations (SDs), supporting the presence of diffuse MM bone disease. Parathyroid hormone levels were depressed and the CT scan of the neck was negative for parathyroid adenomas, excluding a more typical cause of severe and painful diffuse bone disease.

Whilst we were all puzzled by the data before us, the patient suffered a second attack of acute pain in the right seventh rib. An MRI now confirmed the presence of an expansile lesion in the posterior part of the rib. A rib resection (partial removal of the diseased rib) was immediately performed and the histology revealed a plasmacytoma (plasma cell tumor)[f] with no Ig heavy chain (IgH) or Ig LC secretion, i.e. it was a non-secretory plasma cell tumor. Further MRI scans and a second BM examination were yet again negative. It was difficult to make the diagnosis because the diagnostic criteria were not fulfilled. However, even though the only known lesion, the cancerous rib was removed, he continued to have extremely severe symptoms, and not treating him would simply be inhumane.

I therefore made the final decision to treat him as a very non-typical (atypical) case of MM. I decided to individualize his treatment and to avoid chemotherapy for as long as it was possible. A non-cytotoxic (i.e. targeted therapies) regimen was commenced and within three hours his pain subsided. And in two days, he was

---

[e] The globulin or Ig fraction in MM is typically monoclonal (i.e. M-protein or M-band). In inflammatory or reactive processes, e.g. infections, a polyclonal Ig fraction may be found.

[f] Multiple myeloma cells are cancerous plasma cells. A plasma cell tumor or plasmacytoma can exist as a single lesion or as multiple lesions. When present as a single lesion, it is called a solitary plasmacytoma; and when present as multiple lesions, the diagnosis is MM.

Introduction 7

pain-free! After six months of therapy (two months in and out of hospital, and four months as an outpatient), he was in total clinical remission and able to perform all his daily activities. The osteopenia and high polyclonal Igs had both resolved. Interestingly, the initial Hb of 18.0 g/dL (high normal) had decreased to about 13.0 g/dL after treatment. Repeated BM examinations continued to be negative for MM. Today, he remains well after completing eight cycles of targeted therapies that are specific for MM. Could MM be a collection of more diseases than one?

Chapter **2**

DIAGNOSTIC DILEMMAS

"There has to be more than one disease."

Shortfalls of Clinical Criteria for the Diagnosis of MM

Unfortunately, there are no symptoms that are specific for the diagnosis of MM, and interestingly, many patients with MM may have no symptoms at all for a long, long time (years). Hence, in the early stages of the disease, it is often the case that neither the patient nor the doctor knows that this is in fact MM. Consequently, when patients are finally referred to the hematologist, they are frequently already in the more clinically advanced stages (e.g. Salmon-Durie stage IIIA[1]) of MM. Bone pain is the commonest symptom and occurs in about two-thirds of patients. However, it is not a reliable diagnostic criterion because significant MM bone disease is known to occur without the pateint suffering from any symptoms of bone pain. Accordingly, the diagnosis of MM is heavily dependent on laboratory data, including those that characterize MM-related organ dysfunctions. These diagnostic criteria have recently been more clearly defined by the International MM Working Group.[2,3] However, like all things in this world, not everyone agrees to these and either more general or stringent alternative criteria have been proposed, e.g. those from the MM Research Foundation (MMRF).[4] In addition, there is a greater and greater (and almost frenzied) reliance on more sophisticated laboratory testing, which will certainly redefine (and potentially improve on) these criteria further. Modern gene micro-array techniques for gene expression profiling (GEP) have not only separated malignant from non-malignant plasma cell disorders, they have also reclassified MM into newer prognostic groups.[5] The technology is very impressive and will certainly hit the shelves in the future, albeit at a price. And with greater costs comes greater opportunities, which will certainly be different to different patients. Without a doubt, these factors will redefine our abilities and decisions in individualizing treatment for MM patients in the years to come.

"Treat" or "Don't Treat" Diagnostic Grid

One of the favorite diagnostic grids in MM is the almost Shakespearean, "Treat" or "Don't Treat" dogma that is based on a patient's symptoms. Consider the basis for this. If treatment (i) does not guarantee any reasonable level of success; (ii) permanently introduces potentially injurious events; and (iii) potentially makes things irreversibly worse; then it is best not to treat. "If it ain't broke, why fix it?" There is wisdom in waiting until there is good evidence to do things. As doctors, we have been indoctrinated (please forgive the pun) from our formative years of medical education to act wisely and patiently, and to embrace "masterly inactivity" at these most crucial moments in time. When we cannot fix it, it is best then that we do not make it worse. Doctors all have the urge to be decisive and to nip things in the bud; but greater wisdom must be exercised when evidence is thin, and experiment and/or mere experience dictate so (Table 2.1).

I would like to digress a little at this point of time to address briefly the issues of experiential, experimental and evidence-based medicine, and the application (execution) of the evidence in the treatment of patients. As doctors, we sometimes make a unique observation and this stirs up our curiosity and better still, creativity. However, many of these ideas never go any further because clinical research is an arduous task. Hence, experiential medicine frequently stops mid-way in the mental or thought part of experimental medicine. Even if we go further and

10　*Towards Individualized Therapy for Multiple Myeloma*

Table 2.1. Experience, Experiment, Evidence and Execution

	Description	Remarks
Experience	Observation	A doctor frequently begins the journey of enquiry as to the basis of his observation of clinical events through an experience. A lot of this depends on the astuteness of the observer (doctor).
Experimental	Hypothesis	Using his creativity, he proceeds forward along this journey to formulate research hypotheses. Sometimes he will conduct pilot experiments to strengthen his ideas.
Evidence*	Study	Through very complex and controlled processes, clinical trials provide the platforms for testing out these hypotheses in a peer-reviewed setting. The final evidence can be positive or negative.
Execution	Application	Armed with medical evidence, patients can now be treated. It is worthwhile noting that patients, whose profiles would then have excluded them from study, can now receive this treatment.

*So-called evidence-based medicine or EBM.

develop hypotheses, many of these never ever get tested, because it is a huge, huge job requiring tons of resources and funds (sponsorship) to actually conduct a clinical trial. Accordingly, evidence-based medicine or commonly known as EBM, represents only a fraction of all the experience, observation, ideas, creativity and hope that could possibly be conjured up by the human mind. The remaining ideas literally go

---

[g] This is largely true for most experiences. However, there are medical treatments available in the world that have developed without having gone through the rigor of clinical trials. Not all institutions embrace the same dogma as the traditional academic institutions that we know of. Some institutions that conduct modern and sophisticated medical research, in fact, do not subscribe to the convention of peer review and clinical testing. Hence, there's more than meets the eye. But more importantly, is what's lying beneath potentially better, even though relatively unknown? I challenge the reader to consider this strongly because there could be gems out there that never get tested, peer reviewed or published.

into thin air.[g] For those ideas that eventually get tested and, if conducted in the right fashion, they produce positive data; medical practice (in the era of hospital accreditations and standardizations) permits them to be put almost unquestioned into practice. Yes, both doctors and patients rely heavily on EBM. And this is done at the expense of other regimens that could potentially be better but have thus been incarcerated within the contexts of experience and/or experiment. On the extreme downside, it is almost like a "James Bond" movie, where EBM is used as a licence to apply (or execute) treatment to a greater population of patients. This is because during the clinical trial, only certain patients are eligible for study. The others who fall outside the eligibility criteria are excluded from the study group. Once the evidence is obtained (i.e. after the clinical trial), doctors are given the "licence" to use the regimen in all patients regardless of whether they resemble the study group or not. In other words, selectivity is now removed and one size is made to fit all. And if you extrapolate this argument further, EBM and individualization of therapy are in fact very, very different.

Let me elaborate. Data generated from clinical trials is really only representative of a particular sample of patients who fit certain eligibility criteria. It is not uncommon practice, after clinical trial results are published, to extrapolate this and treat patients who are in fact in the non-eligible group. The jury is out as to what constitutes the best medical practices, but one thing is for sure, clinical trials and EBM are extremely biased practices with data that should be taken with a good lump of salt. In the case of MM, virtually every clinical trial excludes patients that do not have a measurable disease using specific parameters. This is obvious; how can one conduct a study on a patient if there is nothing to measure? So, patients with no measurable disease, who might respond extremely well or poorly, and thereby pull results in either direction, are perpetually excluded. Conversely, when EBM regimens are applied to treat patients with no measurable disease, how does one measure response in these patients? There is an obvious system failure which I believe many renowned physicians will agree wholeheartedly with me. We have simply got to find a better way of testing treatments that will make a difference to our patients.

Table 2.2A. The Basis for a Diagnostic Grid based on whether to Treat

	No Symptoms	Symptoms
Insufficient Diagnostic Criteria	Don't treat	Treat
Diagnostic Criteria Met	Don't treat	Treat

Table 2.2B. "Treat" or "Don't Treat" Grid

	No Symptoms	Symptoms
Insufficient Diagnostic Criteria	MGUS Don't treat	?*
Diagnostic Criteria Met	Asymptomatic MM (AMM) Don't treat	MM Treat

*Some have proposed to call these patients early MM (EMM) and to treat them in the same way as for MM.

With these thoughts, let us now address the "Treat" or "Don't Treat" grid (Tables 2.2A and 2.2B) that forms the basis of the way we diagnose and approach the management of MM. As mentioned above, MM is a totally diverse bag of disorders. Genetic analyses have identified at least seven different groups (containing further subgroups) of MM variants.[6] If the diagnosis of MM were as straightforward as the binary code, we wouldn't have a problem recommending treatment even at the earliest instance. Unfortunately, identical genetic signatures are detectable in both asymptomatic, minimally-positive patients with monoclonal gammopathy of undetermined significance (MGUS), as well as patients with full-blown MM. Moreover, patients with aggressive MM may not have any detectable genetic abnormalities, as compared with adverse gene signatures that could be present in the very much silent patient with MGUS. Together, these data suggest that even though we have detected clear genetic groups and subgroups of MM, the impact of these genetic events on MM might be influenced by other factors, or worse, might potentially be totally irrelevant in the clinical setting.

With that rather long preamble about recognizing that MM is actually more diseases than one, it almost feels entirely inappropriate to now squeeze all these possible diagnoses of MM into a 2-by-2 grid (Tables 2.2A and 2.2B). The reader will be somewhat more challenged here because I will be making my arguments from a more philosophical point of view. This is necessary because there is a change that is required, and the change involves the mindset. So let's return to the question of confining MM to a 2-by-2 diagnostic and treatment grid. Firstly, we must understand that we do this because we have not established any consensus on whether MGUS and/or asymptomatic MM (AMM) should or should not be treated. "If it ain't broke, why fix it?" But here comes the challenging part, i.e. if we have new drugs and laboratory assays to support our treatments, why not try to fix it? Consider these scenarios:

- Scenario 1: Old ways, old tools — in *status quo*.
- Scenario 2: Old ways, new tools — get the same results more efficiently.
- Scenario 3: New ways, old tools — getting there slowly but surely.
- Scenario 4: New ways, new tools — way to go!

So, assuming that old ways are inferior to newer methods, then, if we continue to use the old grid (way) and drive treatment using new drugs and laboratory assays (tools), we are in fact using Scenario 2 to treat our patients. We wouldn't have improved on treatment outcome, just getting really good at producing the same results. This is not meant to alarm anyone but to increase our awareness that unless we have new changes to the way we approach this grid, we will not get any further. The experience and experimentation must now be converted to evidence and application (execution) to improve on this diagnostic and treatment grid.

When selecting therapy for the purposes of individualizing treatment, we must be aware that a favorable outcome could require us to consider other, perhaps more critical, factors. Even

14 *Towards Individualized Therapy for Multiple Myeloma*

Table 2.3.   A Proposed Improvement of the Diagnostic-Treatment Grid

	No Symptoms	Symptoms
Insufficient Diagnostic Criteria	MGUS If treatment reverses diagnostic criteria, treat	EMM If treatment improves symptoms, treat
Diagnostic Criteria Met	AMM If treatment reverses diagnostic criteria, treat	MM Treat

though patients do not have symptoms (Table 2.3), they certainly have abnormalities, some of which are touching the very core of life, our DNA. If treatment is able to reverse these abnormalities that constitute the diagnostic criteria for these groups of patients (MGUS and AMM), then these patients logically should be treated. Accordingly, when selecting therapies and assessing response to treatment, our new tools (drugs and laboratory assays) must address the core issues in both pathogenesis (disease causation) as well as cancer biology (i.e. sustenance of deranged and cancerous cellular processes). In addition, it is well-known that certain subjects will fall out of the grid if restricted to 3 squares — MGUS, AMM and MM. In other words, patients with minimal laboratory criteria could have huge clinical problems that require treatment. Failing to treat these patients with so-called EMM could result in grave clinical consequences. Hence, it is the opinion of the author, that patients with EMM should also be treated, especially if treatment improves symptoms. Currently, there is no absolute consensus whether patients with the EMM complex are MM or not. It is precisely because of this that these patients have become one of the biggest challenges to individualized therapy (see Case 3 above).

Prognostic Criteria

Prognostic risk refers to the predicted outcome of a particular patient based on this risk profile at the time of assessment. Diagnosis and prognosis are fundamental to the selection of suitable and relevant treatments. Because the diagnostic grid for MM involves a decision of whether treatment should be commenced, it is not difficult to understand the importance of these prognostic criteria in impacting the decision-making process for therapy. Unfortunately, this is a complicated subject and much data is lacking. Hence, I will not discuss this in detail but will instead provide a simplified risk-adapted treatment grid that I have used frequently in the clinic to conceptualize the salient points. This grid is one of the instruments that can help individualize treatment for patients. It provides a very effective bird's eye view of the disease status, and if performed serially, can provide useful information on the progress of treatment.

The International Staging System (ISS)[7] is currently the most popular and widely-accepted system for assessing the prognosis of MM. Data pooled from more than 10 000 subjects was used to devise the ISS. From the numerous candidate parameters that could be used to assess prognostic risk, only two were consistently significant — the serum albumin and beta-2-microglobulin (B2M) (Table 2.4). One of the features of ISS is the fairly even distribution of cases between the three stages. The effect of this is the assignment of equal weightage for each stage, a very important point for clinical application and trials. Unfortunately, this has compromised the effect of other parameters that are thought to exert an effect on risk stratification, treatment and prognosis. These parameters include, for example, C-reactive protein (CRP) levels, lactate dehydrogenase (LDH) levels, peripheral blood (PB) absolute monocyte counts (AMCO), and most importantly, genetic abnormalities.

Table 2.4. Summary of the ISS Staging System

ISS Stage	Albumin	B2M
I	≥ 35 g/L	≤ 3.5 mg/L
II	< 35 g/L	3.5 to 5.5 mg/L
III	< 35 g/L	> 5.5 mg/L

Significance of Genetic Signatures

As mentioned above, the ISS system very prominently excludes the prognostic significance of genetic abnormalities. Given the amount of laboratory and clinical evidence that has been generated, it is difficult to imagine how genetic signatures do not play an important role in determining prognosis and response of MM to treatment. This has been one of the most controversial aspects of the management of MM today. Patients with particular gene signatures respond differently to certain forms of treatment, e.g. autologous hematopoietic stem cell transplantation (AHSCT). Accordingly, in my decision-making grid, I have included low, medium and high risk categories (Fig. 2.1) that are based on genetic abnormalities, to give practical importance to at least the more established gene signatures:

- Low risk — $t(11;14)$, hyperdiploidy
- Medium risk — normal

0	ISS Stage I	ISS Stage II	ISS Stage III
Low Risk	1	2	3
Medium Risk	4	5	6
High Risk	7	8	9

Figure 2.1.   Decision-making diagnosis-prognosis grid.

- High risk — $t(4;14)$, other IgH (14q32) translocations, hypodiploidy, del(13), p53 mutations/deletions, complex karyotypes.

This composite grid of ISS and genetic categories can now be used, logically, to better understand, prognosticate and plan risk-adapted therapy. Accordingly, Boxes 1 through 9 can now be completed with a sensible set of treatment "commandments" (Fig. 2.2), such as:

- Since tumor burden increases with the ISS stage, patients with stage II disease may require more cycles of treatment than those with stage I disease; and those with stage III disease may require more cycles of treatment than those with stage II disease.
- Prolonged intensive treatment may be required for ISS stage II/III high-risk patients.

Single agent Indefinitely	ISS Stage I	ISS Stage II	ISS Stage III
Low Risk	~6 cycles 1st line +/- Bortezomib AHSCT at relapse	~8 cycles 1st line +/- Bortezomib AHSCT at relapse	~10 cycles 1st line +/- Bortezomib AHSCT at relapse
Medium Risk	~6 cycles 1st line Bortezomib 2nd line AHSCT at relapse	~8 cycles 1st line Bortezomib 2nd line AHSCT at relapse	~10 cycles 1st line Bortezomib 2nd line AHSCT at relapse
High Risk	~6 cycles 1st line Bortezomib 2nd line Novel agents	~4 cycles 1st line Bortezomib 2nd line Novel agents	~2 cycles 1st line Bortezomib 2nd line Novel agents

Figure 2.2. Simple risk-adapted treatment grid.

18   *Towards Individualized Therapy for Multiple Myeloma*

- Patients may choose to reserve AHSCT for managing relapses rather than to have it performed after they achieve complete response (CR).
- High-risk patients should NOT undergo AHSCT if possible.
- High-risk patients should NOT linger too long (e.g. 2 cycles) in a regimen that seemingly does not produce the desired response.
- An important drug for the treatment of MM called bortezomib (Velcade)[8–10] is known to be effective for patients with high prognostic risk gene signatures, and should be considered early.
- Use of novel agents (e.g. in clinical trials) should be considered for ISS stage II/III high-risk patients.

I must stress that this simple risk-adapted treatment grid is to be used ONLY as a guideline. Its strength is its relative simplicity in providing a very succinct overview of the general direction to proceed. Further individualization will need to be done and I will come back to this grid and discuss it further in the book. It is important to be aware that in the course of time, as more information and newer compounds come into practice, the contents of this grid will certainly require a review. Till then, I hope that this grid, presented like a snapshot in time, will help provide you with the concepts of individualized treatment. It is my hope that you will use and modify this grid to suit your clinical practices and/or your treatment plans, for the betterment of therapeutic outcomes for MM.

The 10th Box

You would have noticed that there is also a 10th box, which is numbered "0" (Fig. 2.1). This was not included simply to take up the last space in the grid. It was deliberately designed as a motivational tool, to help patients understand that they may at times have a detectable disease with so little disease burden that full treatment might not be necessary. For example, patients with serum albumin $\geq$ 40 g/L plus B2M < 2.0 mg/L plus normal karyotype. Treatment for such patients could be tailed-down to single agent regimens (Fig. 2.2). During the course of treatment, patients are challenged to attain the 10th box. I will discuss how to convert patients from full regimens to single agent regimens later in the book.

Chapter **3**

SHORTCOMINGS OF MODERN-DAY CLINICAL TRIALS

"Logical extrapolation of medical evidence is badly needed."

Time and again, one hears of others complaining about the difficulty of applying evidence-based clinical trial data to the day-to-day management of patients. In fact, it is sometimes quite amusing to see very prominent and established clinical researchers publicly complaining about their own clinical trials and data. I admire these individuals for their honesty which demonstrates their passion for improving the care and welfare of their patients at the expense of their own reputation. Indeed, the fact that they are the first to complain shows how they have put the patients first. The crux of the matter is that we conduct clinical trials today in a very rigid environment in order to obtain irrefutable evidence that what we are doing is both right and better. Let us not be naïve; the motives behind many of these studies that are done today are driven by manufacturers of drugs who need to establish the use of their products in the market. At first glance, the biases are reasonably obvious. But this is not entirely wrong because newer therapies are very much needed, and clinical trials need to be conducted to bring them into practice. However, I think the problem lies with the fact that institutions continue to confine medical evidence to a box and not permit logical extrapolation to a wider group of patients who

20

obviously will benefit from the extended knowledge from clinical trials. I agree that for the purposes of conducting and controlling the study, the study cohort (or sample) of patients must be made as homogenous as possible. However, that patient sample is for all intents and purposes, a sample. There are many, many more patients who are not in the sample that need treatment. To reach such patients, some customization or individualization of the original protocol is needed. The issue is not that we need to do it, but how this is done as a logical extrapolation of the evidence that was established through rigorous testing.

How Conclusions are Made in Clinical Trials

The fundamental goal of any clinical trial is very simple, i.e. to arrive at a logical conclusion. This is sometimes easier said than done because novel and important findings often defy logic. In its stripped-down barest form, there are two issues (parameters) that need to be reconciled — evidence and correlation. The investigator then has to take three steps to get the answers:

Step 1: Obtain the evidence for each of the two issues.
Step 2: Derive the correlation between the two issues.
Step 3: Assign the importance of the correlation.

Using these 3 steps to guide our conclusions, there could be six possible scenarios (Table 3.1).

- **Scenario 1: Negative Study.** In a negative study, nothing important was found. Hence, there is nothing to correlate with. This can only be true if the clinical trial was conducted at the

Table 3.1.   Concluding Clinical Trial Findings

	Nothing Important	Something Important
No correlation	1 – Negative study	2 – Deficient study
Correlation made	3 – Red herring	4 – Ideal
Over-read results	5 – Taking us for a ride	6 – Too good to be true

required level of performance. Obviously, false negative data will totally mask positive results and one must always be on guard for this. Consider this situation: in many MM clinical trials, as well as clinical trials in other diseases, drug manufacturers and study investigators will exclude patients with poor kidney function from study. If a drug is exceptionally effective in treating MM patients with kidney complications, this drug will never be tested on these patients who are likely to benefit the most. The study would be expected to return with a negative result as it would not be analyzed further for efficacy in the group that is most likely to benefit.

- **Scenario 2: Deficient Study.** In this second scenario, finding positive data for a particular hypothesis is just the first step; making the right conclusion is equally important. Unfortunately, conclusions are only as good as the initial hypotheses that were made. We must realize that hypotheses are colored by numerous shades of differences. If we fail to recognize this, even when obvious shades are present, we could be seeing only stark black and white, and have difficulty in arriving at conclusions. For example, let us say we are interested in the ability of a particular drug to heal bones in MM patients. If we then perform serial X-rays and find that bone lesions are getting smaller and fewer, we quickly conclude that bone formation is a property of this drug. However, we know very well that bone healing is a balance between bone loss and bone formation. Hence, bone healing might just be related to prevention of bone loss and have nothing at all to do with bone formation, i.e. bone formation is occurring indirectly and the drug might not work in patients in whom bone formation is also impaired.

- **Scenario 3: Red Herring.** This is not an uncommon scenario but one to be wary of. Again, our ability to make conclusions depends greatly on the initial hypotheses that we made. In certain situations, nothing related was actually found but yet a correlation could be made due to the way we fashioned our hypothesis. Consider this; thalidomide was tested in a group of MM patients with relapsed/refractory disease. More than 50%

of the patients developed low white cell numbers and as a result, we concluded that this was an adverse effect of thalidomide. If we were able to accurately test BM reserves before thalidomide was given, some patients could have already had critically low levels of white cell precursors. These patients could develop low white cell numbers over a period of time, i.e. regardless of any treatment. In other words, thalidomide might not be a contributory factor at all.

- **Scenario 4: Ideal.** This is the easiest to understand. Some important findings were made and the right correlations lead to positive results.

- **Scenario 5: Taking Us for a Ride.** Of all the scenarios, this is the most worrisome. There is no positive data and yet a strong conclusion was made. In the most innocent of situations, the investigator has accidentally over-interpreted the data and is unaware that he's been taken for a ride. However at the other end of the spectrum, i.e. in the most scandalous of situations, there is complete fabrication of both data and conclusions to the extent of misleading both the medical fraternity and public. Unfortunately, some of these cases have been prominently exposed by the media in recent years. This kind of fabrication of data must be shunned by all.

- **Scenario 6: Too Good to be True.** There is a tendency for youthful researchers to make claims beyond their appropriate measure. Fortunately, in the international peer-review system, "helped" today by the internet, these are also rare but certainly not unlikely events. In the field of MM, there is much color in the dynamics and context of diagnosis and treatment of patients. It is not fair to bring up any example for illustration because there are 10 different apples and another 10 varieties of oranges in the basket. Realistically, we cannot accurately compare and contrast these. However, I actually consider this scenario as one where true medical advances might be found. No doubt, peer-review and time will eventually separate the fakes from the real McCoys. The onus is upon true pioneers to continue to defend their position and ultimately leave behind their legacies.

Assessing Responses — Determining the Context

In my opinion, the Achilles' heel of the management of MM today is our great difficulty in determining treatment responses. Response criteria[11] have evolved over the years with greater and greater emphasis on more and more sensitive laboratory tests. Consider these three types of patients who are not uncommonly encountered in clinical practice.

- There are patients who had seemingly responded well previously, but who had surprised us with sudden, rapid and unexplainable deterioration in their clinical and laboratory parameters.
- And *vice versa*, there are patients who had appeared for all intents-and-purposes to have the worst kinds of MM, but who had made dramatic strides forward on the road to recovery, to the point that they are considered "cured."
- Moreover, there are the all-too-familiar patients in "plateau" phase, in which the status of the disease, determined by the conventional methods that we measure response (e.g. serum protein electrophoresis for an M-protein) today, are neither getting better or worse.

These three types of patients (who are not uncommonly encountered in the clinic) tell us, quite literally, that we are missing something in the way we assess treatment responses. In fact, we seem to admit our failure even in the way we diagnose MM. The prime example are patients who are found to have an M-protein (the so-called condition termed a monoclonal "gammopathy"), and in whom other criteria (clinical and laboratory) are lacking for making a definitive diagnosis of MM. These patients are simply called monoclonal gammopathy of UNDETERMINED significance (MGUS). Whatever the gurus might say, it is my opinion that we really have a serious problem defining responses to therapy in MM. We have placed so much emphasis on the level of the

M-protein, yet the behavior of the disease in certain patients with MM clearly does not correlate with M-protein levels. Moreover, the system simply falls apart in patients who have myelomas that produce no M-protein whatsoever — then what do we do? When you extrapolate the dynamics of the situation further, whatever testing we can realistically do (e.g. weekly blood tests), those data are but snapshots in time that need to be quilted together in order for us to decipher their hidden meaning, much like Egyptian hiero-glyphics. I risk being called a skeptic here, but if I may ask for an honest show of hands, how many of us are able to read hiero-glyphics? The task is a phenomenal one, and we don't even read the language sometimes.

Whilst we are striving to improve our tools of assessment, we have been bombarded by a whole slew of new technologies, includ-ing gene arrays and positron emission technology (PET) scanners. Whether these will turn out as hype or hope is anyone's guess. I should not be read as being a wet blanket here; but rather as truly advocating more research or else how are we to know any better. What I am highlighting is the need for a reality check as well as a deeper insight into the context of the case. Perhaps one of the most nebulous concepts in MM is the so-called "plateau" phase, a state where clinical disease is rather stable and yet there is a persistent and unchanging M-protein level, i.e. stable and detectable disease. It is a term that I find very difficult to apply because it gives one a false sense of security. Consider a patient who was very sick with fever, weight loss, severe bone pain and in whom a fair number of malignant plasma cells had been detected in the BM. Unfortunately, the M-protein level is only marginally elevated. Whilst it should be easy to diagnose MM, the hematologist may be jittery about (i) the accuracy of the diagnosis; (ii) the possibility that the tumor did not produce Igs well; and (iii) the possibility that there could be more than one clone — including one/some that secrete and one/ some that don't. Genetic analyses were performed and they con-firmed gene signatures that were typical of MM. Accordingly, the confidence level that the patient has MM goes up, and the patient commences therapy. Treatment is smooth and by all clinical and laboratory criteria (except the M-protein level), she achieves a remission. Despite the return of BM plasma cells to normal levels, and the clearance of abnormal gene signatures, the M-protein remains unchanged from that at the time of diagnosis. If a hematologist were to see this patient for the first time, he/she might have even diagnosed MGUS and not MM. By conventional criteria, this case would have been considered a non-responder who has achieved a plateau phase.

But what do the context and dynamics of this case really suggest? Has it become MM in plateau phase, MGUS or both? Where do we go from here? Well, I don't have the answers but the context clearly supports a diagnosis of MM at the time of presentation, which was perhaps non-secretory, that was subsequently eradicated by appropriate treatment. However, it was also likely that MGUS, the secreted component, was also present, since MGUS is not really MM but a predisposing plasma cell dyscrasia. The residual MGUS component could have been unaffected or stabilized by seemingly appropriate treatment. However, it continues to remain detectable, much like indelible ink. So, according to recommendations for both plateau phase and MGUS, treatment was gradually tailed-off and lo and behold, the M-protein started to climb again, albeit very slowly. Obviously, this patient needs further assessment for us to fully understand the context of the disease. And we cannot make logical therapeutic decisions if we cannot understand the context of the disease.

Understanding the Dynamics — Key to Individualized Therapy

The key to individualizing therapy in MM is the understanding of the GROUP DYNAMICS that are constantly changing critical parameters in the patient (Fig. 3.1). These include:

- Patient compliance problems
- Multiple myeloma — disease dynamics
- Current treatment options
- Opportunities for novel therapies in the future

Shortcomings of Modern-Day Clinical Trials   27

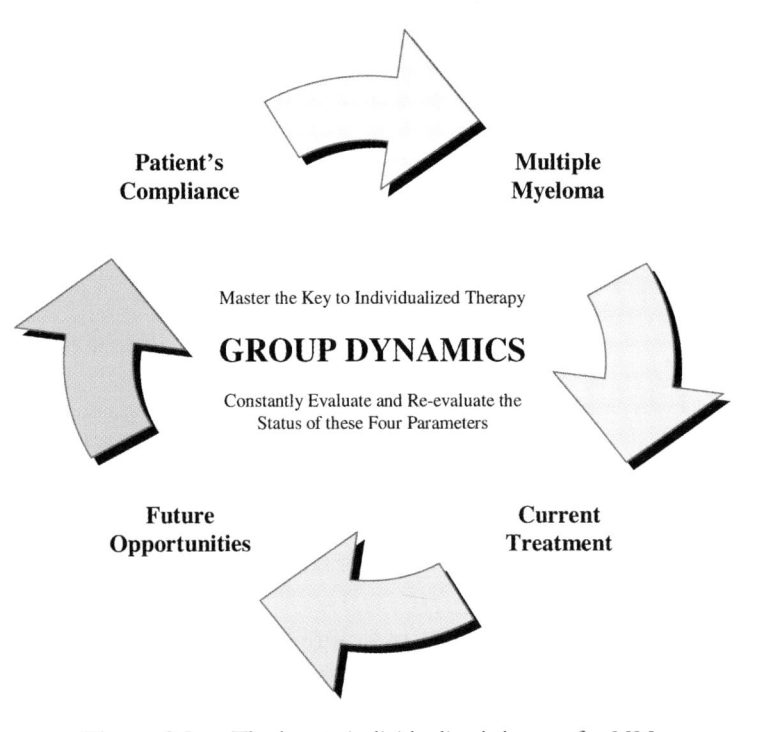

Figure 3.1.   The key to individualized therapy for MM.

Perhaps the best analogy for this is the Rubik's cube. You might have a tough time solving the cube because you really have limited tools. In fact, all the tools that you have are (i) data as snapshots in time; (ii) a risk-adapted treatment grid; (iii) an immensely fallible clinical trials process; and (iv) inadequate diagnostic, prognostic and response criteria; for a mixed bag of conditions called multiple myeloma. These in themselves present significant challenges and controversies. In order to individualize you will need to face up to these challenges and controversies, whilst at the same time juggling at least 16 moving points, all at the same time. And do it with finesse, please!

Chapter **4**

INDIVIDUALIZING CORE PARAMETERS

"Triangular pyramids are amongst the most stable structures."

On March 31st 2008, the Los Angeles Times published a story entitled, "*Let patients weigh in on treatment decisions. Sometimes it's important to get past the protocols and 'rules' to find an approach that's best for everyone.*" In the article, we are reminded that the patient's body belongs to the patient and no one else. We have to respect that. There might be data and rigid regimens all around, but the individual wants therapy individualized for him/her. If we do not value the patient as an individual, we have basically lost our respect for life altogether.

Four Core Parameters

Let's first examine the four core parameters that move together in concert as a group. In this relationship, one parameter cannot change without affecting the others. The point to note is that these are just the core parameters. There is a second layer of sub parameters that further define the core parameters. When we juggle any of these sub parameters in the second layer, the core parameters will also change. Since there are 4 sub parameters for each core parameter, there are in fact a total of 16 sub parameters that we will need to keep an eye out for.

1. *Patient's Compliance*

In my 20 plus years of treating MM, I am totally convinced, without any hesitation, that the single most important factor which leads to successful treatment outcome is the patient's COMPLIANCE. You can lead a horse to water, but you cannot make him drink. Human nature is such that we must first feel motivated deep within us to help ourselves or else nothing will help. It will come as no surprise to leaders, supervisors, CEOs and anyone else in value chain, that success and failure are all about attitude. It's the same with patients with MM. Which is also why, I'm such a skeptic when it comes to accepting data from clinical trials. No-where in any medical journal have I found major clinical trials measuring the attitude and motivation of patients who participate in clinical trials. In fact, this information is so cryptic and the topic so taboo that you sometimes do not even get answers from investigators when you broach on the subject. It is only in the board room, when you have a no-holds-barred meeting that you learn that the attitude of patients can greatly influence the quality of data. Sure we have biostatisticians and the superduperest computer for biometrics analysis. But if we do not have the co-operation of the patient, things can just fall flat. And yes, the biostatisticians do perform some patch-up work, but ultimately what we have is data presented "within statistical limits"; which some of us do not really understand the real significance of, but interestingly, imbibe as gospel truth.

It is not a fallacy that patients do exceptionally well when they are motivated. Sometimes we can "flog" them a little to bring out hidden "talent." But by-and-large, if they want to be cured, they are already halfway there; and if they do not want to, they're (pardon me) as good as half dead. This is not the same as a patient who lacks insight and is unable to grasp the deeper meanings and respond with motivation. A patient who is unable to understand that he needs to be motivated to work towards a certain goal can be exceptionally difficult to treat. In many instances, neither patient nor doctor is able to define clear objectives for the treatment, or set up realistic expectations. And it gets worse when there are preconceived misconceptions. At that point, I nearly always give up. As a doctor, I have no jurisdiction over life and death, furthermore in a patient who wants to live his/her own life his/her own way. And I do respect that. Yes, some patients start off very well. But if the long and winding road is too insurmountable, they behave as humans do and consider taking the short cut down the hill. Such patients are the most challenging ones with the most heart-breaking stories. Sometimes you win them back, but sometimes you lose. To stay motivated, patients must constantly value and love their own lives. And they need to be in control of their bodies. They must feel special to themselves, their families, their friends, their doctor(s) and nurses, and everyone around them. I have never seen a single patient with MM who wants to go through the journey alone. Every single patient wants to have someone with him/her. For the very lonely, this is usually the doctor and the nurses.

I will use the extreme example above to make a valuable point. For such a patient, if the doctor is able to INDIVIDUALIZE (personalize) treatment for him or her, you can see smiles like stars and galaxies orbiting in the room. In my practice, where we focus on individualizing every patient's treatment, I have never ever had a patient who rejected our attempts at tailoring treatment to his/her needs, be it medical, social, economic/financial or even plain old practical and common sense. When faced with a disease like cancer, the patient knows that the problem for all intents and purposes is his/hers and his/hers alone. So when the doctor is able to fashion treatment to suit his/her environment, such that he/she is totally comfortable with it, this patient will feel as if he/she has managed to co-opt another to share his/her burden in the most personal way, and the journey is no longer a lonely and arduous one. Doctors and nurses, and even family, friends, employer, church members etc, who go that extra mile for this patient would have done the most important thing, and that is to motivate him/her to get cured.

So then, what are the key areas that need constant balancing? There are four fundamental areas:

- The patient's overall health.
- His/her immediate social supports — family and friends.
- His/her personal motivation.
- His/her tolerance to treatment and will to be cured.

With individualized treatment, the compliance meter goes up by leaps and bounds. When patients remain compliant, the sky is the limit; you can do almost anything with and for them. There is no doubt that compliance leads to improved treatment outcome. In a small pilot study that I conducted on MM patients, all patients who were non-compliant fell below the line; and all those who were compliant at least 80% of the time, rose above their non-compliant counterparts. And this has been my consistent experience with subsequent patients. I have a label for these patients, who are compliant, and in whom we are able to individualize treatment. This label is "Optimal." Optimal treatment, to me, is not just delivering the drugs at the target doses. I am a firm believer of the "80/20 Principle." Optimal treatment to me is achieving at least 80% of the target dose of medicines, AND being able to individualize at least 80% of the confounding factors that surround that patient. In reality, you frequently never achieve 100% of the target dose of medicine. However, if you only do this (i.e. achieve 100% of the target dose) and neglect the other 15 balance points, your patient will literally lose his/her balance and fall off.

The age-old saying is true, "one size doesn't fit all." Do not expect to do the same thing for each patient. The "one size fit all" phenomenon only happens in (not the movies) the clinical trials. I hope I have made my point clear enough. Do not expect it to happen like in the clinical trials (the "movies") unless you are the actor/actress. Patients do not have the luxury of splicing scenes. For them, the movie starts and ends without a break, and they have to deal with it, day in and day out. So do not blame them if they lose the will to fight on, it isn't an easy journey at all. If doctors and nurses continue to expect patients to clear every obstacle in front of them, or worse still, placing more obstacles before the patients and expecting them to just leap over, can anyone blame the patients if they lose their motivation and become poorly compliant. So we need to be flexible. Get a few sizes in to try. Pick the one that fits best before going home with it. We all know how to do that when we go to the stores. It's the same with treatment. We need to give our patients a whole rack of sizes to try.

Now imagine incorporating flexibility into a tightly regulated healthcare system, e.g. the government/federal hospitals. It actually becomes very difficult. In the end, both patient and doctor become frustrated; sometimes to the point of giving up. When hospitals engage themselves in benchmarking exercises, the problem actually escalates. Numerous accreditation exercises for hospitals may in fact work against the interests of both patients and doctors. I am not writing this as part of a blame game. We must all understand that this is one of the directions that healthcare systems are embracing today. At the risk of sounding like a cliché, it's just part of the system we're all caught in. Healthcare systems after all do not work for the individual but for the common good of the whole. The difficult parts are the grey areas where system rigidity must give way to flexibility. Figure 4.1 is an example of an artificial and, honestly, relatively rigid grid. (*Grids are always rigid; I use them but never really liked them.*) But give it some color, as in Fig. 4.2, and permit the color to change with time, and now we see how flexibility can be built into a system that now has some nice layers. From a matrix, we now have a Rubik's cube. Here things change constantly and yet remain inseparably together. The game is to solve it without breaking the cube apart or replacing the color tabs. Sometimes you win; sometimes you do not and become so frustrated. Sometimes the patient scrambles it, and you try to solve it. Sometimes you inadvertently scramble it further. Sometimes the patient begins to solve it, and on the other hand, you are trying your best to scramble it, and so you're both back to square

Individualizing Core Parameters   33

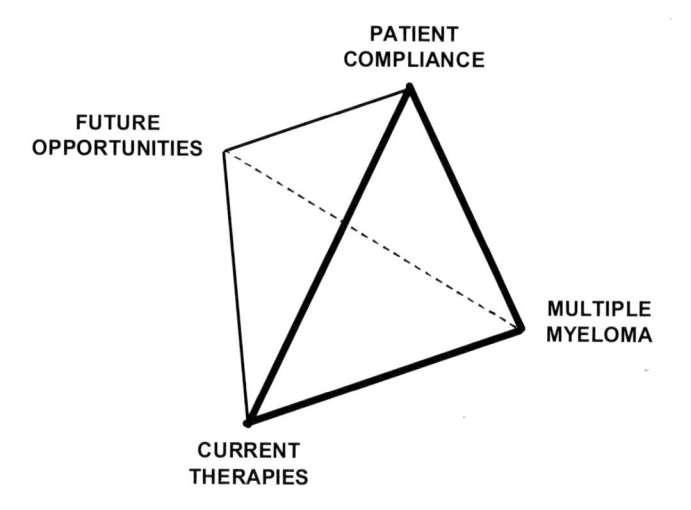

Figure 4.1.   Four core parameters — triangular pyramid.

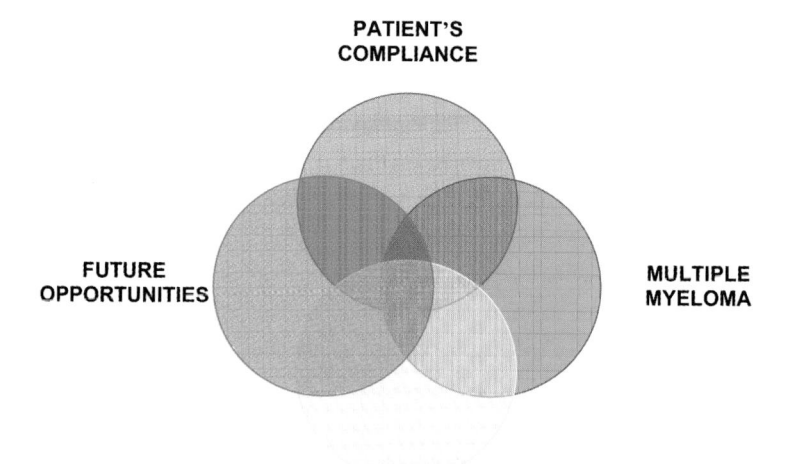

Figure 4.2.   Four core parameters — Venn diagram.

one. But try and try again. Ultimately both of you will solve it together.

2. *Multiple Myeloma*

If one considers MM to be specific to a patient, one is in fact referring to the subtype of MM that the patient has. MM is traditionally categorized into subtypes according to the common type of monoclonal Ig or Ab the whole population of cancerous MM cells secrete. Whilst this has provided us with a working framework for many years, in reality the disease processes that make these cells cancerous are far more complicated and involve even non-cancerous cells. In the simplest terms, MM cells do not survive in the body alone and unaided; they survive in a nice home on a comfortable bed that is actually provided by the host. The normal cells provide and protect these cancer cells, almost like hypnotized slaves. The uncanny ability of fugitive MM cells to survive and grow in this host environment, away from surveillance by the immune system is possible because MM cells are masters of disguise and expert con artistes. They are also highly capable underworld crooks that worm their way into the ranks of the protectors and engage critical help and services from the immune system itself in order to evade and flourish in the body. Dramatic as this may sound, these events actually happen in the body. Unless we recognize the extent of the deception they create, we cannot possibly fathom the dire consequences should we become complacent and let down our guard during treatment. There are four processes that need to be balanced within this section on the disease, these are:

- MM — the disease itself.
- The BM microenvironment — the so-called tumor bed.
- The blood supply — the nutrients and especially the cells that perpetuate the cancerous processes.
- The immune system — how the body attacks the cancer cells internally.

Individualizing Core Parameters   35

Before going further, we must first recognize that the organ of the body that MM originates from is the immune system. In other words, MM is a cancer of the immune system. Specifically, MM is a cancer of the Ab (or liquid; non-cellular) form of immunity. The non-cancerous normal counterpart of the MM cell is that cell that produces Abs (proteinaceous substances) in our immune system, the plasma cell. This is in contrast to cellular immunity where immune system cells actually take part in battles with foreign substances. Interestingly, our body uses these normal immune system cells (immunocytes) to eliminate cancerous cells (including MM cells). But I do not want to confuse you further, and will just summarize and say that MM cells are members of the immune system but with no useful immune function because they are cancerous. They evade detection by normal immunocytes through a wide variety of methods (which are beyond the scope of this book) and in fact seem to live almost like parasites in the body. They know how to do this very well, perhaps because they originate from the immune system itself. Accordingly, MM is one of the hardest cancers to eradicate since drugs that inhibit the MM also inhibit the normal immune system; e.g. chemotherapy. However, newer drugs that specifically target biological pathways in the MM cell that are unique to the cancer cell and less so the normal immune system (e.g. bortezomib or Velcade) have been shown to be exceptionally effective in MM. Hence, these new agents, so-called targeted therapies, bring the hope that not only can we now destroy MM cells, we can also protect and even enhance the remaining immunity at the same time, perhaps to a level whereby we would have a good chance of overcoming the cancerous process. Now that we appreciate, at least broadly, the scheming nature of this disease, let us focus on the process of myelomagenesis — a complex process in itself and refers to the interactions of the four major biological processes that produce and propagate MM.

You might be surprised to know that MM cells are quite fragile. When removed (explanted) from the body and placed in cell culture media inside biological incubators, these cancer cells stop growing almost immediately. By contrast, when you remove normal cells from the body and do the same, i.e. put them in cell culture media and incubate them, they survive for about a week. In fact, normal cells from tissues like the back of the nose (the area called the nasopharynx) or heart will show rhythmic movement when viewed under the microscope, as is their normal function for such movements. In other words, nasopharyngeal cells that bear tiny hair-like projections can be seen to produce very fine and coordinated wave-like movements, and heart cells show rhythmic beating, just like what heart cells should do. Yet, despite the tremendous variety of laboratory tools that we have today to make explanted cells (which have been placed in incubators for cell culture) grow, explanted MM cells simply do not. Their growth stops almost immediately and at times mid-way within cell division. This is a state called the interphase.

One of the tools of modern research in the fields of molecular biology, cellular biology and medicine is the cell line. Cell lines are explanted cells have been kept in continuous cell culture generation after generation. Some of these cells were derived more than 50 years ago from patients who have long since passed on. It is quite amazing that the owners of these cells have already died but have left behind a legacy that is actually living in a tissue culture flask! There are literally hundreds and thousands of cell lines kept in cell line collections in many parts of the world. Whilst the majority of these are cancer cell lines, there are also some normal tissue that have been, as it were immortalized using various methods, e.g. viral infections. And whilst there are for example a hundred or more breast cancer cell lines, for nearly 50 years, there were only two genuine MM cell lines! Simply put, MM cells cannot live outside the human body. They need what is called the tumor bed to survive. Very fastidious.

The tumor bed is not a simple tissue, it is incredibly complex. But it is composed of normal tissue — chiefly supporting cells, non-cellular tissue (called the extracellular matrix or ECM) and blood vessels that bring in nutrition. The normal supporting cells do just what their name suggests, i.e. support, but also can be coerced, as it were, to "join forces" with the MM cells. Join the "dark side" so

Individualizing Core Parameters 37

to speak. One of the most prolific of these evil consorts in MM is the osteoclast (OC). The OC is actually a normal bone cell. Since the main home of MM cells is the BM, bone cells are part of the tumor bed. Accordingly, OCs and another type of bone cell called the osteoblast (OB) are part of this tumor bed. The function of OCs is to remove mineralized (mainly calcium compounds) bone, and the function of OBs is to lay down bone. These two related processes go on continuously in everyone, i.e. normal persons, to ensure bone health. This process is called bone remodeling.

Interestingly, OCs produce a substance called interleukin-6 (IL-6) that is a critical growth factor for MM cells.[12-15] To MM cells, IL-6 is the elixir of life and OCs are the biggest producers of IL-6 in the tumor bed. In order for MM cells to engage OCs to produce IL-6, signals must be sent from one cell to the other, a process that has been termed "cell talk" (intercellular signaling). Cell talk can be achieved through direct cell-to-cell interactions or indirectly through messenger substances between cells. When "talking" is direct, the forward messaging signal on the surface of the "talking" cell, called a ligand, must meet a receptor on the surface of the other "listening" cell. And to "talk back," the receptor-ligand relationships reverse direction, usually through another pair of cell surface molecules. Of these two processes, direct cell-to-cell receptor-ligand "cell talk" is by far the most efficient and indicates an absolute dependence by each cell on the other. Cell-to-cell interactions are most critical in the tumor bed. It's as if the cancer is now fully-integrated (100%) with the surrounding normal tissue where it lives and thrives and is protected, just as if it were normal. This is a difficult concept to understand but it is the foremost element to consider when individualizing treatment for patients with MM. One must recognize that the MM development process, i.e. myelomagenesis, is one of absolute (100%) deception to the extent that the cancer looks for all intents and purposes normal to the body's immune system. You can even call it parasitism. So when we treat patients with MM, we need to go right down to the tumor bed to break the bonds between normal and cancer. We need to separate the normal from the parasites.

To compound matters, OCs are but one of the cells that MM cells require in the tumor bed. There are other supporting cells, including fibrous cells (called fibroblasts) as well as scavenger cells (called macrophages). Fibroblasts also secrete ECM, which is like scaffolding tissue in the tumor bed. And then there are blood vessels and the blood cells, oxygen and nutrients that come in blood. It is beyond the scope of this book to discuss in detail all the complex interactions. However, one of the blood cells that are exceptionally important are the monocytes. I will elaborate more on the monocytes later in the book. For now, the important concepts to note are:

- There is a huge amount of cell talk going on.
- There is even cell talk from non-cellular ECM matrix.
- Cell talk communicates with blood vessel cells to bring in more blood (including monocytes), oxygen and nutrients via a process called angiogenesis.
- Blood vessels provide a highway for MM cells to escape to other places and spread via a process called metastasis.
- Blood vessels also bring in the immune system and medicines that can rid MM cells from the body.

Perhaps the most sinister of all the biological processes is not the MM-OC interaction, or angiogenesis. It is the body's inability to identify and fight off MM cells, i.e. the failure of our immune system to recognize cancer. Every person produces cancer cells each day. It is estimated that there could be as many as a thousand a day. Yet we do not develop a thousand cancers a day, we do not even develop a thousand a month, or a year, or a lifetime. What happened to these cancer cells? Well, most of them died naturally through a built-in process called programmed cell death (apoptosis). But some certainly survived and if given the right environment, would seed and germinate. Our immune system is thought to function like policemen, looking out for these crooks and removing them from the streets. The process is called host tumor immunosurveillance. Somehow this has broken down

Individualizing Core Parameters   39

and one of these MM crooks had escaped and found an underground alliance with OCs and the rest of the tumor bed. Broadly, there are four basic ways that MM cells can evade the immune system:

- The MM cell disguises and becomes invisible by lowering (downregulating) cell surface markers that the immune system uses to identify these cells as cancerous.
- The MM cell inhibits the access and mobility (cell migration) of the immune system cells so that they cannot catch up and the MM cell runs away.
- The MM cell inhibits the function of the immune system so that even if it identifies the MM cell, it cannot kill it via a process called immunoparesis.
- The MM cell inhibits the growth or even kills the immune system cell, via the secretion of inhibitory molecules.

Actually, the MM cell is even "smarter" in that it uses the activated immune system to grow even faster. And this is a real lesson in group dynamics. Consider this paradox: if failure of host tumor immunosurveillance was the original event that permitted seeding and growth of MM cells, then one would expect that if all things remained the same (which they usually do not), then continued failure of host tumor immunosurveillance would propagate MM more and more. Yes, logical. In events that broadly activate the immune system, e.g. infections, one would expect to see some tumor regression, as is the case of using bacillus Calmet-Guerin (BCG) vaccinations to treat bladder cancer. However, one of the most frequent observations in MM is the intense flare-up of MM, to the point of disease progression and/or relapse in patients who encounter infections. The activation of immune function leads to the growth of MM cells. In essence, the group dynamics have changed when MM establishes itself in its home. It is actually capable of using signals from activated immunocytes called T lymphocytes/cells to grow and undergo mutations. The reason for this is that the normal counterparts of MM cells, i.e. the plasma cells, use these T cell

40 Towards Individualized Therapy for Multiple Myeloma

Table 4.1. Group Dynamics Analysis of MM Treatment Strategies

	Worst Scenario	Treatment Strategy
MM Cell	Genetic mutations	Attack MM strongly
OC	Absolute parasitism	Attack OC strongly
Angiogenesis	Double-edged sword	Moderate inhibition
Immune system	Double-edged sword	Permit recovery to normal Suppress over-activation

signals (especially receptor-ligand signal called CD40-CD40 ligand (CD40L)) to perform DNA mutational events and burst cell growth as a phenomenon of the normal immune response. The three points to appreciate are: (i) MM cells use their normal in-laid biological processes for this; (ii) it is not evasion of the immune system but coercion; and (iii) the event is an explosive one.

In Table 4.1, you can see that the group dynamics in the realm of MM biology is an extremely complex one. On the one hand, we need to augment the immune system, but on the other hand, an activated immune system actually triggers an explosion of MM cell growth. We need to reduce cancer-related blood vessel growth or angiogenesis. Yet at the same time, by doing so, we reduce our ability to deliver drugs to kill MM cells and hamper the reparative processes that are mediated by the immune system. The concept of moderation or "less is more" is exemplified in the treatment of MM using drugs that target angiogenesis as well as those that inhibit or activate the immune system. In contrast, the use of anti-MM and anti-OC medicines, as well as drugs that can deal with high-risk genetic signatures (by removing and/or preventing gene mutations) should be pushed to its limits.

3. Current Treatment

There is much debate on what is current treatment for MM. This includes international summits and organizations devoted just to determine the evidence for recommending specific treatment regimens. The National Cancer Care Network (NCCN)[16] is such an

Individualizing Core Parameters   41

agency that has published clear guidelines for physicians to use. Yet, differences in geographical location and healthcare systems will dictate how much one can adhere to these guidelines. It is therefore more fruitful to look at the broader concepts that guide the way we approach therapy, rather than the regimens themselves. There is no point in discussing high-dose chemotherapy in a country that does not have resources to treat infections. Rather, it is better to consider the realistic group dynamics that govern therapy as we experience it today.

Let us first consider the impact of age of presentation of MM. In the figure (Fig. 4.3), let Time = 0 be the point at which diagnosis was first diagnosed. The observation period is 120 months or 10 years. If most cases of MM present between ages 40 years and 70 years, we can create a mathematical model for the overall survival of all persons at the limits defined by the age of presentation. Hence, persons who are age 40 years at the point of entry, are not expected to die over the next 10 years, and their mathematically modeled survival curve can be found at the top (-▲-). By contrast, persons who are age 70 years at the point of entry are generally not expected to live much longer and many would have

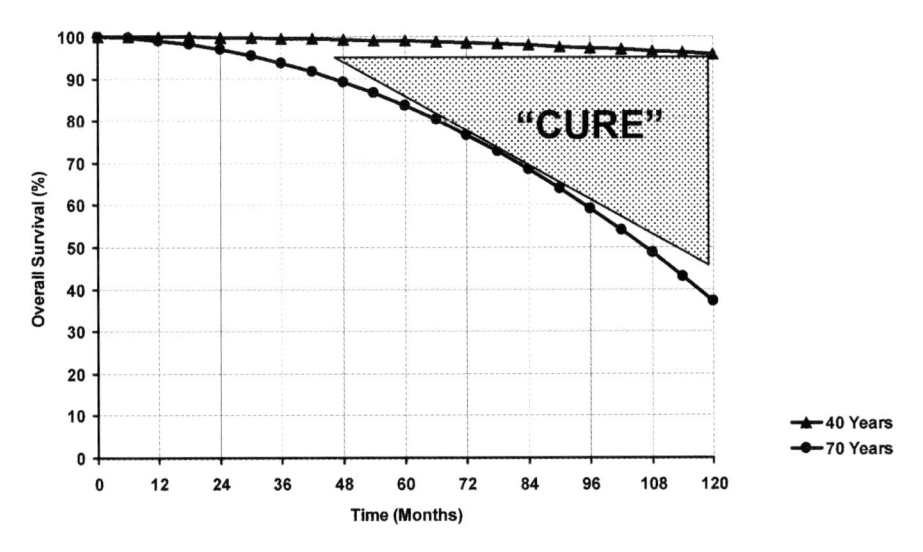

Figure 4.3.   The triangle in the corner — "cure".

42   *Towards Individualized Therapy for Multiple Myeloma*

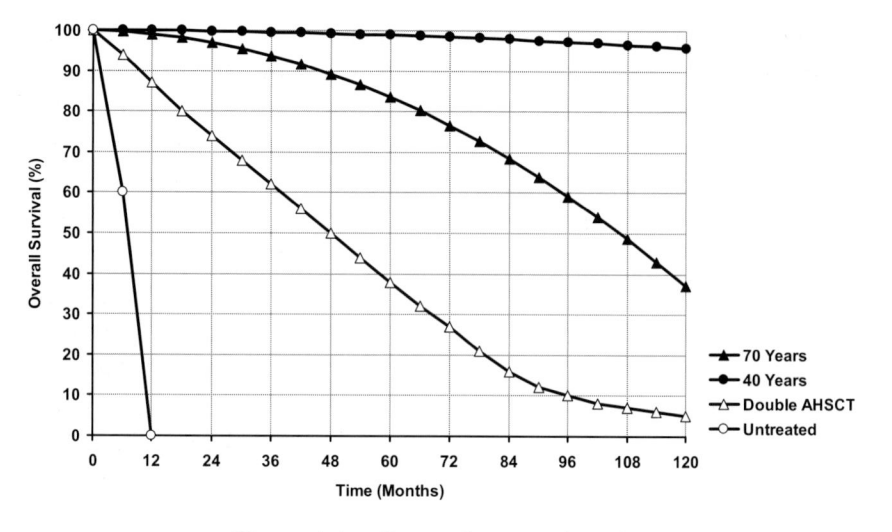

Figure 4.4. Status of current therapies.

died within the next 10 years. If we assume that about two-thirds of the cohort of persons at age 70 years will die before 80 years, then the mathematically modeled survival curve will be the lower one (-●-). The curved triangle in the top right hand corner is the mathematically modeled expected survival of patients who otherwise do not have MM. It also represents the goal of therapy, i.e. if we can make the survival curves from treatment fall within the triangle in the corner, then we would have achieved a functional "cure."

If we now mathematically model patients of whatever age (mostly 40 year olds to 70 year olds) who were either untreated (-○-) or treated with the best recommended regimens today, e.g. double AHSCT (-△-), we can now see the status of our present treatments (Fig. 4.4). The data speaks for itself, results are dismal. Even with double AHSCT, we are barely halfway towards "cure." Granted, there have been great improvements from the time when patients were left very much untreated. However, after more than 50 years of attempts at curing MM, we are still nowhere near "cure." Most of the 50–60 years have been devoted to the development of chemotherapy-based regimens. In fact, AHSCT is for all intents and purposes high-dose chemotherapy followed by rescue

Individualizing Core Parameters 43

using the patient's own stem cells. Despite these mega doses of chemotherapy, there have been really very few, if any, "cures." These possibly "cured" patients from high-dose chemotherapy followed by AHSCT can be seen at the 10-year mark where the graph appears to rise above the zero percent (0%) level. However, beyond 10 years, even this seemingly optimistic data is lost as the graph creeps back down to zero.

One of the points to note about double AHSCT in MM is it is frequently a planned procedure right from the time of presentation. In the recommended treatment algorithm of the 1990s and early 2000s, round about the time when double AHSCT was in vogue, AHSCT, whether single or double, was built right into this algorithm as a planned procedure which followed a number of cycles of conventional chemotherapy (Fig. 4.5). What is not usually mentioned is that the amount of chemotherapy actually given is quite massive; about 5-fold to 10-fold conventional doses. Moreover, before the first AHSCT, there is a round of high-dose chemotherapy (usually a drug called cyclophosphamide), which is given to release (mobilize) stem cells from the BM for collection from the PB through a procedure called apheresis. Should the

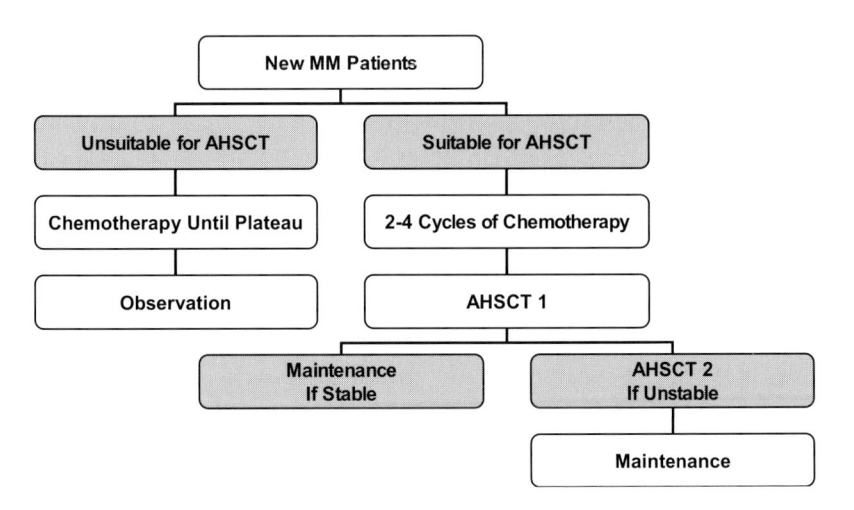

Figure 4.5. Treatment algorithm for MM in the 1990s and early 2000s.

patient require the second AHSCT and the first stem cell collection was inadequate, in principle, the patient could undergo a second cyclophosphamide mobilization followed by HSCT collection and the second transplant.

Hence, in the extreme scenario, the patient from the time of diagnosis would have undergone four rounds of conventional chemotherapy; two rounds of chemotherapy mobilization; and two rounds of high-dose chemotherapy followed by two rounds of autologous transplants. This is equivalent to about 20 cycles or more of conventional chemotherapy and the patient is expected to survive all that. The rewards are survivals as noted in Fig. 4B and 100% grade 3 or grade 4 toxicity, and a real, real risk of treatment-related mortality (death from treatment). Unfortunately, the hope for cure is for all intents and purposes, very, very close to ZERO. It is interesting to note that MM is the cancer in which the highest total doses of chemotherapy are planned as treatment for the patient right from day 1; and this is done with the knowledge that there is practically no chance of long-term cure. Clearly, chemotherapy is not the way forward for MM and that something new is required.

Unfortunately or fortunately, depending on whether you are an advocate or opponent of stem cell transplantation, the majority of patients do not qualify for transplantation. Currently, AHSCT is only recommended for younger (below 65 years of age) patients because of the toxicities related to high-dose chemotherapy. Attempts to reduce the dose of chemotherapy for transplants in those above the age of 65 years have generally shown no survival benefit and greater treatment-related toxicity. Hence, the general consensus is that AHSCT is not recommended for those over 65 years of age. Accordingly, a good one-third or more patients are immediately excluded from the mega chemotherapy arm of the algorithm. For the remaining two-thirds of patients, many will have co-morbidities like kidney failure and heart disease that could make high-dose chemotherapy and AHSCT difficult. Others who qualify for AHSCT on the basis of medical assessment might not be able to produce enough stem cells after mobilization. Still others would refuse AHSCT for whatever reasons. In the end, depending on the medical centre treating patients with MM, the percentage of patients finally eligible for AHSCT could only be around 10% to 25%. Then there are centers that do not perform AHSCT at all because of limited resources or taboos. The global figure for AHSCT is, as I predict only about 10%. This means that conventional chemotherapy still forms the bread and butter of treatment for many patients.

So, coming back to our mathematical model (Fig. 4.6), I have now added two forms of conventional chemotherapy, melphalan + prednisolone (MP) (- -▲- -), and vincristine + adriamycin + dexamethasone (VAD) (- -●- -). You can immediately appreciate that they do not perform as well as double AHSCT. The area within the curves for MP and VAD represent the outcome of current treatment for MM for about 90% of patients in the world. There are only 1 conclusion and 1 action required and those are — MM has not been conquered and more research is needed. From experience, to experiment, to evidence and finally to application, without hesitation, patients with MM need to see more of this.

The incidence of MM in Asia is between 1:100 000 and 2:100 000, and in the western countries about 4:100 000. Because of the general lack of resources, many MM patients in Asia might

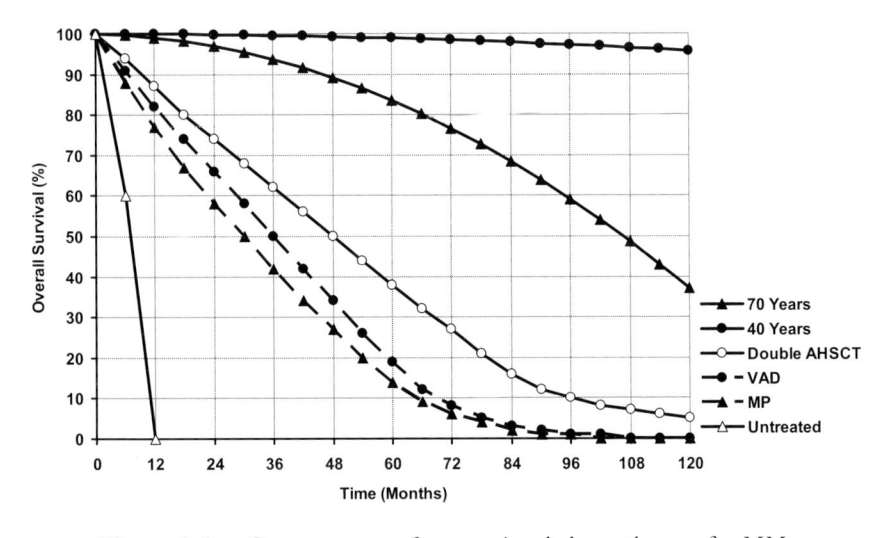

Figure 4.6. Current status of conventional chemotherapy for MM.

not get diagnosed. If we assume that the true incidence of MM in Asia is 2:100 000; and 80% of the world's population are in Asia, then there are twice (i.e. half the incidence but four-fold the population in Asia as compared to western countries) as many Asian patients with MM as there are in western countries. The burden of finding a cure for MM is definitely on Asia. Hence, when considering the group dynamics for successful treatment of MM, regimens that are suitable for Asian patients should take top priority in the pursuit of "cure" for MM. If pharmaceutical companies are serious in addressing the needs of MM patients in a global context, they need to study and understand the Asian patient with MM. The Asian patient is the individual who will make up half, if not more, of the burden of MM in the future. He/she is the individual whose treatment needs to be individualized.

4. *Future Opportunities*

The future certainly will lie not in the hands of the patient, but in the hands of the researchers, drug manufacturers, investors and regulators (Table 4.2). Each of these has a critical role to play and vital obstacles to clear. There will be a tendency to develop newer compounds with as wide a reach as possible, a product that is doubtfully suitable in all patients. The hope will be that there will be sufficient varieties to swatch (mix and match) to suit every individual. At the end of the day, the responsibility of swatching will rest on the doctor and his patient. Treatment outcome will depend almost certainly on who is treating who.

Table 4.2.   Here Lies the Future

	Critical Role	Critical Obstacle
Academic sponsors (Including researchers)	New compounds	Bureaucracy
Pharmaceutical sponsors	Clinical trials	Let clinicians lead
Commercial sponsors (Investors)	Catalyst	Sustain interest
Health regulators	Safety & Affordability	Exercise flexibility

Our observations from the experiences of AHSCT have taught us some valuable lessons. Chiefly, that MM cells are by nature (whatever the mechanism) resistant to chemotherapy. More is not more; perhaps less is more; or none is best. Bad news for pharmaceutical companies that have put in gazillions into funding chemotherapy research. Sad news for those who were treated unsuccessfully. But we mustn't make this a blame game. Rather we must pick up from where we left off and learn quickly from our mistakes. At no time has it become more important for us to listen to the individual patient than now. It is really not too late to stop the rhetoric and start listening. If we cannot hope to get rid of all MM cells, why not aim to keep tumor burden as low as possible, and give patients an excellent quality of life. After all, for patients who first develop MM at 70 years of age, individual happiness might in reality be the obvious goal of all therapy. Bringing tumor burden to as low as possible in as comfortable a manner as can be achieved might be the most desirable avenue to take.

We need new compounds that heal and yet not do more damage. We need compounds that make patients comfortable and happy during treatment. We need fewer injections, longer dosing intervals, fewer undesirable side effects, etc. We need more researchers to find them. The problem with academia is, very bluntly, red tape and bureaucracy. There is an alarmingly high rate of frustration amongst the very bright persons that are doing the legwork in our laboratories, because of bureaucracy. The case in point is made in the cloning of the human genome, where commercially-driven enterprise outstripped academia at such a blistering pace, that the final outcome was almost laughable.

But just finding new compounds is not enough, we need them in the clinics and we need to see results in real patients. This responsibility has traditionally been left to the pharmaceutical sponsors, who will no doubt develop programs that are rewarding to their companies first, before patients. If more is more, all the more better. However, sarcasms aside, pharmaceutical companies have come of age and in certain instances, have recognized the useful synergy to let clinicians take the lead. I consider this a very important step forward in that for the first time, we will have the resources to lead clinical studies that address the individual needs of patients. The so-called investigator-initiated trials or studies (IIT/IIS) are the way forward in bridging the gap between the drugs and the patient.

Effective Individualized Treatment Regimens for MM can only Arise from Clinical Research Studies Performed in the Format of IITs.

Probably the most conflicting parameter in this equation is the role of the external, third-party investor. In a nutshell, there is a conflict of interest and integrity issue. The problem with share-holders is their impatience for quick returns. A good drug can have the carpet pulled right under its feet by "uncaring" investors. Sustainability of investments will permit development of good drugs with high margins of return, but only if investors can recognize that there is usually a very long lead time for research and development. This actually becomes compounded because in trying to solve the long gaps, investors insist on stacking up pipeline compounds for concurrent development. The problem is, there aren't enough of these to go around and we end up developing products that are of little benefit or use, or do not solve the problem, or makes things worse. This is a difficult issue because there is a lot of money involved usually and board decisions do not always consider the needs of the patient.

A final word on health regulators who must ensure safety of all drugs (this is not to be compromised), as well as ensure affordability (this is debatable). I do not think there is much to fault their existence, otherwise there is little to ensure that we do justice to our patients. The only point that needs to be stressed is that in their enthusiasm to ensure the best for the whole healthcare system, there is a tendency towards undue rigidity. Some flexibility is required, even at the highest echelons of the health ministry. Patients deserve safe drugs but not deprivation in the face of life and death; after all, no one lives for that patient. He/she is an individual needing individualized treatment.

Chapter 5

PATIENT COMPLIANCE

"Myeloma cannot be eradicated in a non-compliant patient."

The key sub parameters that relate to a patient's compliance are (Fig. 5.1):

- His/her health
- His/her family and friends
- His/her tolerance to treatment and self will
- His/her resources

1. The Patient's Health

Of the four chief sub parameters, health is the most personal. In order to deliver individualized therapy, patients with MM should be concerned about their own health. If they are not, they are responding inappropriately and definitely need help from family members, friends or anyone else (e.g. social workers, support groups). Patients going through the grief reaction may display denial or aggression, which lead to indifference or stubbornness, respectively. On the other hand, patients who are coping well after the grief reaction, frequently display constant personal attention to their health and well-being of their bodies. Those who are more physically capable and motivated may include regular workouts to

49

50   *Towards Individualized Therapy for Multiple Myeloma*

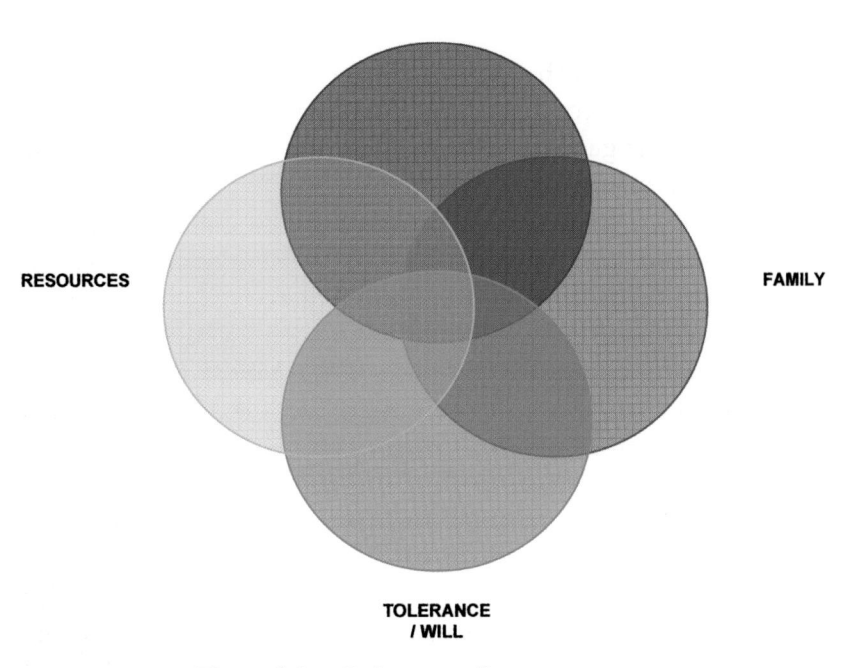

Figure 5.1.   Patient compliance parameters.

enhance the anti-tumor functions of their immune systems. Recent anecdotal reports appear to suggest that one could work off cancer through extremely strenuous exercises, e.g. climbing mountains. I am not suggesting that these are true, but certainly, if you are a patient and want to try it out, there are many mountains that are just waiting to be scaled.

In a motivated patient, compliance is usually not a problem. He/she can be relied on to be vigilant about symptoms, medication, side effects management and regular follow-up. Individualizing treatment becomes easy because there is a constant flow of information between him/her and the doctor and nurse. And everything is almost picture perfect; almost. There are three major imperfections that we must recognize, even in these so-called model patients:

- **What lies beneath?** Patients can still develop serious side effects that are totally unexpected. Accordingly, we must not let down our guard despite the seemingly easy passage during therapy. Remember, still waters run deep. What lies beneath may be exceedingly difficult to predict. I recall a patient who was a model patient who eventually died because an accident that was just waiting to happen was brewing right under our noses and we never expected it. This patient was the dream patient who always came on schedule and on time, who followed all the directions from his doctors using a handwritten diary. He even recorded his weight and temperature every day and took daily walks in the park. He was meticulous (but not obsessive) with cleanliness, loved his health and his life. He also loved pineapple juice. Now you might ask what possibly could go wrong with liking pineapple juice. Except that his favorite stall was not in the city but in a more rural area. He would go there ever so often until he was struck with MM and was advised to take food only from hygienic places. But ever since he started to show a good clinical response, he let down his guard and started going to his pineapple juice stall again; and more and more often. Till one day when he inadvertently took pineapple juice from a stall, parked by the side of the road, that was less hygienic. He very quickly developed stomach cramps which worsened at a blistering pace. Without a good immune system, he progressed to portal pyemia (infection of the blood near the liver), massive mesenteric thrombosis (blood clots in the intestine's blood vessel system) and extensive bowel infarction (death of intestines because of stoppage of blood flow). Unfortunately, his life ended in a very tragic manner.

- **Faking it.** I remember this other patient of mine very well. He had a very mild dementia and also a mild Parkinson's disease.[h] But he could be relied upon to always come on time for his appointments and give all of us a big smile. His daughter would come with him at times, whenever she had time off from work. But most of the visits, he was alone for consultations and extremely positive. It was decided one day that he would require intensification of medication as his M-protein level had risen and his hemoglobin had fallen. A higher dose of medicines was prescribed and instructions were given to both the patient and his daughter (by phone). To this new line of therapy, he took enthusiastically (almost euphorically). But we didn't realize till later that he actually didn't understand his medication instructions and was faking it. In the subsequent 3–4 weeks, he was admitted to hospital for recurrent episodes of mild urinary tract infection (UTI), which was attributed to enlargement of his prostate. Then one day, he was admitted to hospital for a severe pneumonia (infection of the lungs) and careful examination of his remaining medicines alerted us to a medication error. He had taken all 3 months of medicine in 3 weeks and had no more medication left. Apparently, he had been so enthusiastic about getting well and the chance of taking more medicines to do this, he interpreted the increased doses as an all-out effort to rid him of his MM, once and for all. Fortunately, he survived and we all learned a good lesson. From henceforth, he was only prescribed medicines with supervision by his daughter, who now became the gatekeeper. And I'm pleased to say that he's doing well with treatment.
- **Mr Smarty Pants.** This last patient of mine is probably an all too familiar one in this age of the internet. The latest bane of

---

[h] Parkinson's disease is a nerve disorder where patients basically have great difficulty initiating movement. When they do succeed, they have difficult moving smoothly and stopping their actions. At rest, they can be seen to have shakes in e.g. the hands and fingers.

medical practice, i.e. patients who come into the clinic loaded stacks of paper carrying the "www" label. It's interesting how nowadays patients and others rely so much on the internet when they should be consulting their doctors instead. Fortunately, "Mr Smarty Pants" is sometimes right. However, unfortunately, he frequently (if not always) doesn't see the whole picture. I will say this categorically, and not just to defend my trade, that one will miss the woods for the trees if one tried to out-smart his/her doctor. When approaching the treatment of a difficult condition, such as cancer, a very broad and open bird's eye view of the whole picture is critical in planning investigations and treatment. Even more so today, when there is so much information overload, there is really a lot of knowledge to integrate before some logical course of action can be formulated and executed. Some of this information are not medical, and could be logistical, administrative, regulatory or even political. Overall, patients still rely greatly on the doctor, but I recall one who didn't. "Mdm Smarty Pants" was a rare and tenacious one. Armed with a pen and not paper, but a personal digital assistant (PDA), she was almost like a political reporter or the paparazzi. Her knowledge was extensive. Her questions very thought provoking. She was masterly in selecting the most comprehensive therapies for her. But her problem was that, she saw a whole board of physicians and quacks. And one day she was admitted into the hospital with what appeared to be an explosive flare up of her MM. Till today, I do not know for sure what happened, but the story goes that she had consulted an herbalist who prescribed a tonic that would stimulate the immune system. It was a kind of pagan immunotherapy. I suspect that the substance she took possibly contained IL-6, the most potent growth factor for MM. So, her MM flared up quite badly. But fortunately, after some months of treatment, she improved but not fully. But have you ever met a leopard who changed its spots? Yes, you've guessed it, she did it again. Her MM flared a second time as an aggressive plasmablastic variant; and this time, nothing could help "Mdm Smarty Pants." A really sad ending because all she wanted was to help herself get well; but perhaps with too much enthusiasm.

Clearly and without a doubt, patients come in all shapes and sizes. Don't kid yourself to think that you can just pluck one of those respectable clinical trials regimens out of the "cookbook" and use it successfully. Before you know it, things need alteration. No doctor who uses a treatment algorithm stays on it without adapting it to the patient's constitution and circumstances. If you want your patients to do well, individualize, individualize and individualize. Get to know them very well, and swatch treatments around until they work. Fixed protocols and regimens are ONLY for the clinical trials. This is the case in point. We conducted a clinical trial using a certain individualized regimen for all comers with relapsed MM and demonstrated responses in two-thirds (65%) of patients. Encouraged by this we did the same clinical trial to a more select group of newly-diagnosed patients — same individualized regimen but now in untreated patients. This time three-quarters (75%) of patients responded. Then we applied our knowledge in real-life setting, permitting individualization of every possible parameter we could think of. The result: nearly 90% responded with the same regimen. This just goes to show that the regimen defined by the clinical trial is only a part of the whole individualization process. For patients to do well, more can be done than just using newer and better drugs. But patients may not do so well if they lack motivation or insight. The inability to work together with the doctor towards a workable treatment schedule because of lack of understanding may lead patients to a poorer therapeutic outcome, in spite of all the best medicines that we have today. Moreover, factors like family members and friends, willpower and resources also come into play.

2. Family

Family members and friends are one of the greatest resources for patients with MM. Unlike other cancers, MM patients rely significantly more on family members, friends, their employers and others for a number of reasons:

- **Pain.** As one of the most painful cancers, many patients with advanced MM depend on help from others, sometimes constantly. Patients with severe bone lesions (especially pathological fractures) need assistance with activities of daily living (ADL), including moving from one place to another (ambulation), brushing their teeth, feeding and bathing. These are things that you and I take for granted; but believe me, MM patients literally struggle with these throughout the day. It is really miserable for them. Medication, sometimes very strong (e.g. morphine and sedatives), can help most patients but bring along a new spectrum of side effects, including constipation, hallucinations and even addiction. These side effects are well-known confounding problems that many MM families go through. In fact, patients themselves know very well that they may succumb to these additional problems if they are not constantly watchful. Addiction to sedatives (e.g. midazolam, Dormicum) can arise surreptitiously in seemingly careful patients. Family members can in fact help patients become addicted if they are easily over-ridden. For example, if the husband-patient is behemothly dominating and the wife-caregiver is bogged down with other family needs, e.g. young children and elderly parents. So how does one individualize therapy in such a situation? It is obvious that these MM families need help, and urgently. No help is too much and too soon. For exanple, individualizing treatment can take the form of intensifying bone healing measures over above what we would normally do. Do not hold back for the lack of good reason; patients need it. Close follow-up is also necessary, as events can change very quickly and very drastically. A lot will depend on the vigilance of the patient and doctor.
- **Peripheral neuropathy (PNY).** From pain, let's now move to an almost painless condition called peripheral neuropathy (PNY). Fortunately, this is not so common. And because it is less common, both doctors and patients often do not recognize

it. As the name suggests, there is an abnormality of the nerves. Although there are a number of mechanisms that can lead to PNY in MM, one of the more well recognized ways is damage to the insulation of nerve fibers (i.e. the so-called myelin sheathe) by M-proteins. Moreover, drugs that are used to treat MM, e.g. thalidomide and bortezomib (Velcade), are well-known to cause PNY.[17] In fact, there are other causes of PNY in MM, and collectively, they make this condition worse in both frequency and amplitude. Although some PNYs can be painful, the majority lead to painlessness or numbness. There is also associated weakness of the muscles that are activated by the affected nerves. And in some of the more severe cases, muscles become very thin and weakness can be profound. In the most severe cases, the muscles that are required for breathing and eye/eyelid movements might also be affected. In these extreme MM patients, treatment in the ICU may also be needed. Such drastic forms of treatment and monitoring could require the use of mechanical ventilation and continuous cardiac monitoring. It is not difficult to imagine the burden and anxiety that will be placed on family members and friends when MM patients are in this life-threatening situation. The decision to abandon all rules and protocols is never clearer than now. The patient who is fighting for his/her life needs 100% individualized therapy. Moreover, he/she needs this on an hour-by-hour, minute-by-minute basis, since deteriorations and improvements in bodily functions can be very rapid. It is also important that the professional medical and nursing team take over management unimpeded by family members and friends, as it is unlikely that the lay-person is qualified to handle any of these problems. The role of the family members and friends is reduced to a vigil, with episodes of consultation by the medical team for issues like consent for investigative procedures. Since PNY is a spectrum from the very least to the most catastrophic, at each stage of severity, varying degrees of individualization should be introduced. Again, one size cannot fit all. Commencing with avoidance of drugs that cause PNY; to using algorithms to allow dosing whilst allowing recovery of PNY; and to the treatment of other causes of PNY (e.g. diabetes mellitus). In any event, MM patients will continue to come in all shapes and sizes, so individualization must be robust, creative and agile.

- **Kidney failure.** The M-protein is actually composed of two types of proteins called light (LC) and heavy (IgH) Ig chains. M-proteins are found dissolved in the aqueous (liquid, water) component of blood and travel to all the organs, including the kidneys. Since the kidneys are filters for blood, the liquid portion of blood passes through the pores of these biological filters. Blood cells and large proteins (e.g. IgH chains) don't normally filter through because of their size. However, Ig LCs pass freely through. Unfortunately, Ig LCs induce damage to tissues when they are present at a high concentration. In this case, kidney cells are damaged, resulting in what is termed, renal (for kidney) impairment. In as much as a third of patients with MM, there is significant renal impairment making treatment difficult. The uniqueness of MM here, as compared to other cancers, is that MM is actually quite remote from the kidney, but yet produces profound renal damage that eventually leads to kidney failure. Patients in this situation require dialysis and with it, all the inconveniences surrounding the complications and logistics of going for dialysis. If they are immobile, e.g. because of pain and fractures, their needs and reliance on family and friends escalate. Accordingly, the burden on the resources of MM families will also escalate. However, with treatment, some MM patients can show significant improvements in renal function, to the point that they do not require any more dialysis. This will certainly be a welcomed relief for family members and friends and constitutes a definite aim of therapy for all patients. Unfortunately, the repertoire of drugs that can be used is very much limited by the presence of poor kidney function. For example, bone active agents, e.g. zoledronic acid, cannot be used because of the side-effect of toxicity on the kidneys (also know as nephrotoxicity). Certain drugs that are cleared by the kidneys (e.g. thalidomide) tend to accumulate in renal failure and doses must be lowered accordingly. In individualizing treatment for such patients who need constant help from the family members and friends (usual caregivers), a list of nephrotoxic drugs as well as renal dialysis schedules must be taken into consideration. Some nephrotoxic drugs can still be given if the doses can be adjusted for the degree of renal impairment. Slower rates of infusion might also aid delivery of drugs that would otherwise be contraindicated because of poor renal function. Since drugs that can be removed by dialysis must not be given just before dialysis, but rather immediately after, creative scheduling of dialysis appointments with treatment cycles can permit both to be done. In this respect, it is worthwhile noting that visiting the MM treatment clinics will now be placed downstream of visits to the dialysis centers in the normal work flow for the day. Hence, patients may only arrive for treatment late in the evening or the following day. In addition, having dialysis earlier (e.g. in the morning) will help family members and friends in their care-giving roles.

- **Recurrent infections.** I remember very well an amazing patient with recurrent infections. Her journey began with a cough which was treated with antibiotics by her general practitioner (GP). Treatment was a little longer than usual because her immunity was depressed (a state that is termed, immunocompromise). Because of this, she developed a very bad diarrhea from the antibiotics. This depressed her immunity and prolonged damage of her intestinal tissue which lead to further infection by a nasty virus that lurks in our body passages, the cytomegalovirus (CMV). We call such an infection by CMV an opportunistic infection. Unfortunately, this was not recognized early as it is a rare type of infection. Her continued immunocompromise lead her to develop one the most amazing infections, CMV infection of the eyes. In this situation, her eyeballs, which contain a jelly-like material became culture chambers for CMV — a horrendous infection. Because CMV eye infections affect the visual functions of the eye by causing inflammation to the eyes (retinitis) and subsequently, blindness, a decision to quickly treat CMV retinitis was made and the patient started on a drug called valganciclovir. One of the side effects of this drug is further immunosuppression and immunocompromise. Accordingly, the patient went into a spiral and developed recurrent bouts of pneumonia. This lead her to develop a chronic infectious lung disorder called bronchiectasis, where lung tissue is severely damaged and converted to pockets of culture media harboring mixtures of organisms, some of which are germs of low importance, but others of very much higher propensity for life-threatening events. The burden of the family members and friends was tremendous, not only for the frequent use of expensive antibiotics and Igs, but also for the prolonged number of days in hospital to complete such treatment. The message on individualizing treatment for such patients is surprisingly simple. Balance the treatment of MM with the preservation and if possible augmentation of the immune system (Table 5.1). Easier said than done because immediately, all chemotherapeutic agents go out of the window along with glucocorticoids (e.g. dexamethasone and Pred). We are then left with a handful of agents that have a variety of anti-MM effects without negative effects on the immune system. These drugs include zoledronic acid, thalidomide and bortezomib. Unfortunately, there is a profound lack of evidence-based data to guide doctors in individualizing treatment in such situations. Specifically, we do not have clear guidelines on how to combine medicines in a logical way to both ensure efficacy and maintain safety. The following grid gives us some insight on how swatching can be done:

Table 5.1. The Basis of Immunoprotective Agents in MM

Drug	Use In	Avoid In
Zometa	Bone problems & most patients	Kidney failure
Thalidomide	Most patients	Liver disease
Velcade	Most patients	Peripheral neuropathy
Immunoglobulins	Active infections & most patients	High blood proteins

So how do we individualize treatment for family members and friends when it comes to recurrent infections in the patient? The most important role for family members and friends is to have a broad idea of what kinds of morbidities and co-morbidities the patient has. This is because older folk who suffer from infections often cannot speak coherently and might not be able to give the doctor a clear account of his/her medical problems. Family members and friends can help by having an individualized record of the main medical problems that the patient has. If the patient has been going for regular dialysis or frequently collecting urine samples for example, the patient could be having kidney failure. In which case, zoledronic acid should not be given. Or if the patient is known to enjoy drinking alcoholic spirits very frequently, thalidomide might not be expected to work except in large doses. Hence, not giving thalidomide to avoid unwanted side effects might be a good idea. Simple but critical information of the individual kept readily available by family members and friends could save lives.

3. Tolerance/Will

I would like to return to the point of the patient's motivation during treatment because this is linked very closely to his tolerance and will to overcome his disease. Also, I will not claim to be a philosopher by any measure, and will write as a doctor and a layman. In doing so, I risk being called an amateur and ask that you bear with my ignorance in this subject. It is because I consider this section very appropriate for management of the patient and the individualization of his/her treatment that I cannot omit it.

As discussed earlier in the book, tolerance, will and motivation are all very personal and vital characteristics of the patient that need to be nursed (if at all possible). Like consciousness, they define areas in a person that are inaccessible to others; that only that person can use or change. No two persons (or patients) are alike psychologically and socially in these areas. Accordingly, there are numerous shades and hues that like a painting make up that individual. But more than being an image that is captured as a snapshot in time, tolerance, will and motivation changes, moment-by-moment. They adapt to changes in the immediate environment (e.g. mood) as well as to more distant or indirect changes such as social, medical, financial changes and other circumstances. The permutations are virtually unlimited and impossible to discuss. What needs to be made aware and emphasized is that we must always be sensitive to the patient in areas that affect his tolerance, will and motivation. Nothing is more difficult to handle than a patient who has lost his/her will to live, who is no more motivated to come for treatment, and who is like this because he or she had great difficulties tolerating treatment. Permit me to illustrate this.

The patient with an IgG MM was a wealthy woman in her sixth decade of her life. She had been having back pain for several months, and was found to have compression fractures in many vertebrae (bones of the spine) on MRI scanning. She had consulted her doctor who recommended starting treatment for MM. Curiously, she refused, despite knowing that she had a cancer and that the cancer had invaded her spine and that she could be paralyzed if disease were not quickly managed. Why had this occurred? Her decision clearly defied commonsense and logical thinking. In choosing to refuse treatment, she had risked a permanent and serious disability. What could make a person accept this fate today, where everything could be available, especially for the wealthy? It turned out that she had been planning a very elaborate vacation that involved several other people. And she had always been the one who looked perfect for the day; the one that rose above her "competitors" victorious. Her motivation was to appear invincible, even in the face of death (quite literally). There was no way she was going to let a "little" cancer beat her. She was going to pulverize it instead by showing up at her party/holiday unfazed by that little blimp that happened a few weeks ago. She would tolerate it till the trip ended and all the dust had settled. She had set her will to do it and there was to be no turning back.

Not unexpectedly, she got to do what she wanted. But what was more important than the events was the context behind these occurrences. You see, she made her mark at the casinos. This was her final game in which she was gambling with her own life. She couldn't pass the thrill of a high-stakes game. The doctors were helpless against her decision and were left aghast. Fortunately, this was not in Copacabana and there wasn't any blood or even a single gun shot. And it was settled quite amicably with all her doctors walking out on her. It's amazing how intensely determined the human spirit can be. The willingness and sheer nerve to risk everything and tolerate everything in the face of danger is fairly admirable, at least for the guts of it all. I guess some of us would go bungee jumping, whereas others would not. What was it that so deeply motivated her?

Alas, the fairy tale ending was not to be. She gambled and lost. Her holiday had to be terminated on the second day. She had slipped, fallen and fractured her spine further. Her body became contorted and she had fainted from the intense pain that accompanied the fall. When she arrived at my clinic, she was a mangled mess that needed an urgent fixing-up. But not without some token protest, which I permitted, since she was entitled to some face-saving dignity. Whilst we worked on getting MM under control, more work had to be done on changing the way she approached her disease — her tolerance, will and motivation were valuable strengths that, if not misdirected or misaligned, could be turned to her advantage. There lay the real challenges.

I will fast-forward events to the end of six cycles of initial (induction) therapy, where a partial response (PR) to treatment was recorded. She was now able to walk with a walking frame but with a rather pronounced curve in her back (a lordosis). She had refused surgery, hardly an unexpected conclusion, and had demonstrated a fair amount of resentment to caregivers, who without reason also bore the brunt of the blame for her state. (Who ever heard of a "good loser" in the casino anyway?) So, we discussed details about subsequent therapy. Surprisingly, she was quite amenable to trying a second, albeit stronger regimen. But not really surprising because treatment had taken the form of a new game where she could wager her life against the odds of success or failure, where she could gamble at the high-stakes table again. In which case, were we now able to redirect her will to getting herself cured? Or was this too good to be true, that she was instead using us as poker chips.

Little did we know that the rest of the story was about to play itself out in the most peculiar way. So, second-line treatment was started using a regimen that had drugs that led to a larger spectrum of side effects. Moreover, many of these side effects were also of greater intensity and tenacity, resulting in substantially more morbidity, a truly bitter pill to take. Did she enjoy it? Not in the least. Did it bring up new problems? A mountain of them. She went through what was essentially an extremely colorful grief reaction, from sadness, to aggression, to bargaining and finally, yes finally, to acceptance. But she could not go one more step to learn to cope with the stress that came along with the grief of the side effects. Without being too revealing, we heard a bucket of lies and cries, as well as an encyclopedia of vulgarities. There were near fist fights, blood and near suicides before calm finally drew in. She was gambling with whatever she had, compromise after compromise. Treatment was mayhem — we didn't know what or who was to be believed. Things became so surreal after a while. How you wished you could restart the level and choose "Easy," just as you would on your X-Box.

In all my years treating of MM, this was really the most difficult patient. There was no way that we knew that could motivate this patient in a positive way. Her absolute intolerance to side effects sparked off like fireworks, events that took ever so long to resolve. When the dust could finally settle, she didn't have the will to fight on and cope with the new changes. We simply could not improve her health because there was no motivation to be compliant with treatment anymore. Sadly, she progressively deteriorated, becoming increasingly emancipated over weeks and months. Her visits to the casino and clinic both dwindled as her resources got more depleted. And then she quite miserably rode off into the sunset...a tragic ending.

4. Resources

Resources are the reality check in individualizing therapy for MM. We can do only as much as we have. But we should do all we can without withholding anything because we would have lost opportunities if we had held back. Some things will not wait for us; some will bring us up to another level; and some will irreversibly change the course of our lives. But if we fail to do as much as we can, we have not capitalized on our available resources. This is the time to cash in the chips because the survival graphs are still far away from the "cure" triangle with standard therapy (Fig. 4.6). With the introduction of the targeted therapies, these trends in patient treatment outcome are set to change. The following are factors to consider when estimating your resources in the face of the increasing availability of modern targeted therapies:

- **Cost of modern targeted therapies.** Many of these new/novel drugs are not inexpensive. However, there is a clear trend towards lower toxicity as compared to approximately equivalent therapies. This translates to substantially lower indirect costs of therapy. When all costs are considered, targeted therapies frequently offer a cheaper form of therapy than e.g. chemotherapy and/or transplantation. Hence, when total costs (and not just the costs of medicines) are factored in, it is possibly wiser to use limited resources on therapies that provide a better cost:benefit ratio, than on treatments where hidden costs lurk in the background.
- **Availability of targeted therapies.** Across the world, not all medical centers are equal. From infrastructure to services; from hygiene to food; and from doctor's training and expertise to experience and confidence; things are simply different. This is certainly true for the targeted therapies. What has been more and more frequently observed is the fact that center to center variation is a significant factor in the outcome of targeted therapies. In a recent review in The Oncologist,[18] in which a total of 18 very similar studies were compared for the treatment of

relapsed/refractory MM, wide variations of response rates (RR) between 39% and 93%, as well as remission rates, between 6% and 64%, were recorded. These differences cannot be fully explained by the differences in the regimens; and cannot exclude the effects of center to center variation. These factors need to be carefully examined in order to make an informed choice and decision. The availability of a larger number of centers that deliver superior targeted therapy programs may on the one hand contribute to a wider net of available resources; but on the other hand put an undue strain on more personal resources, e.g. available funds.

- **Finances and Intangible Resources.** We have discussed some of these earlier, e.g. support from family members and friends, who constitute extraordinary resources. Some of these resources that come with family members and friends are indeed quite intangible, including love, honesty and the more spiritual issues. At the other extreme, I have observed negative elements arising from matters that surround the family, including hatred and betrayal, cheating and fights. In many of these, money and finances have been significant factors. Although the more intangible resources appear to be tucked away in their niche, the reality is they seldom do. All too frequently, they are aligned with issues of costs and finances. Accordingly, I have concluded that modern medicine is unable to separate itself from financial resources. Greater reliance on third party financing (e.g. health insurance) will be amplified in the years to come and we cannot exclude ourselves from this fate of modern mankind.

There are without doubt more wonderfully ramifying scenarios and factors that surround the availability of resources that are available to the patient. Rather than discuss more of these, I would prefer to discuss an approach to individualizing treatment based on the resources available to that individual. First, let us consider the types of resources that are available to the patient at the time of diagnosis.

66   *Towards Individualized Therapy for Multiple Myeloma*

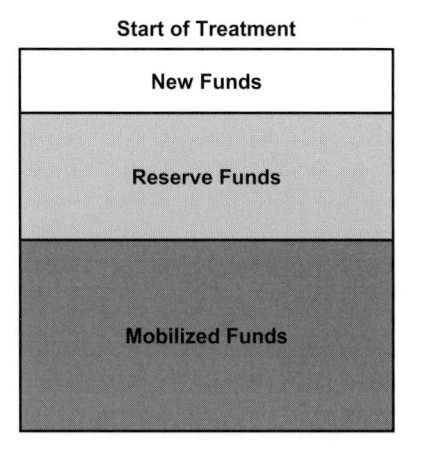

Figure 5.2.   Resources at the time of diagnosis.

At the start of treatment (Fig. 5.2), mobilized funds are the funds that can be used immediately for investigations and treatment. In simple terms, let's consider these as cash and instruments of cash. They usually constitute the bulk of available funds. Patients frequently have reserve funds that can be used on a rainy day, e.g. gold and property that can be sold for cash. They probably constitute a smaller fraction of all the funds. Finally, there could be new funds that are not already available, e.g. donations from family members and friends. These constitute the smallest fraction.

The commonest scenario of resource depletion during treatment is the one where funds are fixed (Fig. 5.3). This greatly reduces the mobilized funds component, putting stress on the patient's reserves funds. After some time, patients could be forced to use reserve funds, thereby triggering alarm bells for the need to acquire new funds; e.g. appeal for donations from loved ones or even the public. Clearly, this is a situation that all patients dread. The reality is it really happens in patients with cancer. Treatment of MM is not always simple and at times expensive (e.g. transplantation). Sometimes patients may be eligible to participate in clinical trials where some or all of the costs of therapy are provided by sponsors (usually pharmaceutical companies that manufacture the

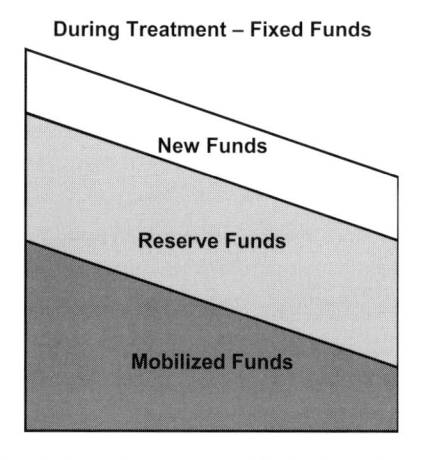

Figure 5.3. Depletion of resources with fixed funds during treatment.

study drugs). In those situations, patients may acquire additional funding of a limited and regulated nature. But if they demonstrate clinical benefit from novel treatment regimens, they become true beneficiaries of the clinical trials process.

The contribution of clinical trials to the patient's resources is depicted by Fig. 5.4. Essentially, mobilized funds have been depleted, but the patient may be able to protect the depletion of reserve funds by participating in clinical trials that provide at least some level of funding, including the use of novel therapeutic agents (e.g. targeted therapies). In studies that are not directly led by pharmaceutical companies, but supported and financed by pharmaceutical companies, i.e. so-called IITs, patients are further protected by institutional research investigators from the undesirable commercial aspects of the clinical trials "business" that are fueled by the pharmaceutical industry. This is because institutional research investigators who run IITs conduct the study in an academic setting rather than from a commercial angle. The scientific questions basically asked are concerned with whether the drug is a good one for the diseases, rather than if the drug is better than a competing one, which elevates its market status. This is a fundamental point because the sponsor, or study chief, is now an academician rather

68   *Towards Individualized Therapy for Multiple Myeloma*

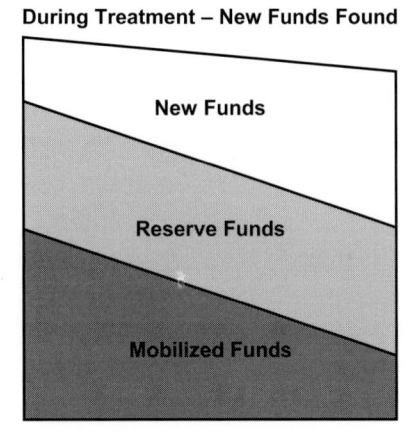

Figure 5.4.   Depletion of resources where new funds are found during treatment.

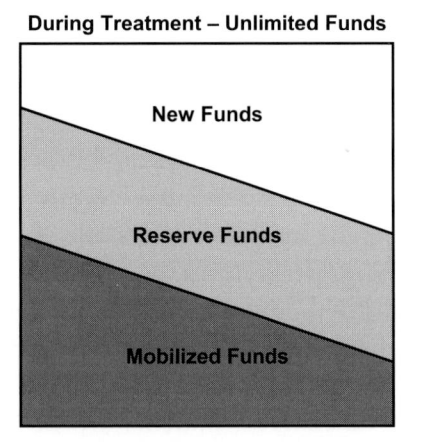

Figure 5.5.   Depletion of resources where unlimited new funds are found during treatment.

than an executive of the corporation. Accordingly, the rights of the patient are better protected by this arrangement.

Of course, if there were unlimited new funds throughout treatment (Fig. 5.5), then the patient continues to benefit from treatment with minimal stress on resources. The situation is akin to

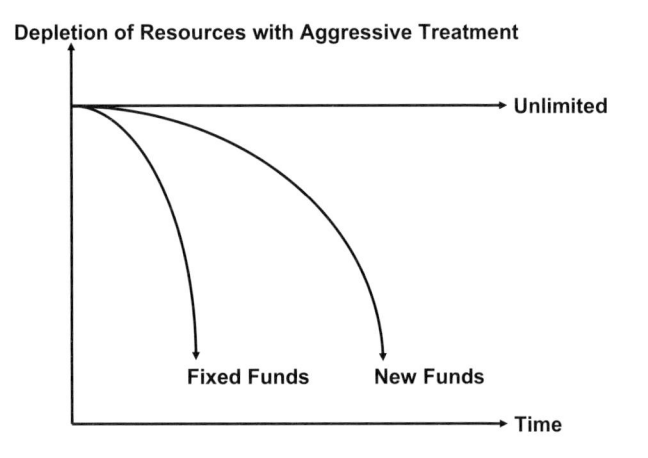

Figure 5.6. Impact of aggressive therapies on resources.

moving from one clinical trial to another, for patients where no other new funding resources are available. The caveat is that there will always be new agents and clinical trials to test them. Hence, this situation might be a hypothetical or an ideal one, and one that might not exist in reality, except for some.

The hypothetical model for the depletion of resources and funds when a patient is placed on an aggressive mode of therapy is shown in Fig. 5.6. Therapies like chemotherapy which come with it the treatment of complications of chemotherapy, e.g. infections requiring hospitalization for antibiotic therapy, can be considered as aggressive forms of therapy that rapidly deplete funds and resources. With fixed funding, it is easy to understand how rapid this process is. Even when new funds are injected, when treatment is aggressive, depletion of funds take a slower but still a relatively steep course. In situations where patients encounter serious consequences that require treatment in ICUs, funds literally vaporize into thin air. This is especially in patients that required repeated invasive interventions, e.g. endoscopy; or repeated imaging procedures, e.g. CT scans; or special procedures, e.g. dialysis. All these contribute to hidden costs that are unplanned and unpredictable. In reality, they add to the risk of the therapy.

70 *Towards Individualized Therapy for Multiple Myeloma*

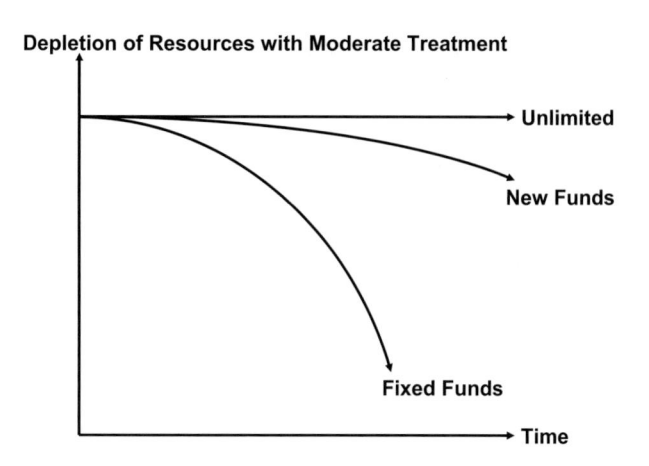

Figure 5.7. Impact of moderate therapies on resources.

When treatment can be moderated to become less aggressive (Fig. 5.7), it is expected that there will be fewer surprises from unpredictable adverse events and unplanned costs. Moderated treatment, e.g. the targeted therapies, promote a fundamental change in the way we approach the treatment of cancer. This is particularly true for MM, where no true cures have been achieved with the amounts of chemotherapy that had been given to patients. In other words, broadly speaking, except for a very small fraction of patients, chemotherapy cannot cure MM. If cure is not possible, and chemotherapy increases morbidity, mortality and costs of treatment, then why not aim, not for cure, but for reduction of tumor burden and improving quality of life. In other words, convert MM to a chronic illness where tumor burden is minimum and there is a low risk of full-blown relapse. And do just that by using treatment that is minimally toxic and sufficiently moderated, so that these patients are not under undue risk of developing adverse side effects. The clinical experience with targeted therapies is precisely like this. That even patients with fixed funds can sustain longer periods of treatment with good quality of life and with a relatively low risk of serious complications. Moreover, many patients can be managed as outpatients, with fewer episodes of hospitalization, let alone treatment in the ICU.

In patients that are able to acquire new funds, e.g. by participation in clinical trials, the graph moves upwards. Such patients, considering the effect of time and aging, might be well supported to live to a ripe old age with sufficient resources to see them through. This is a real and almost ideal situation. Hence, in considering how to individualize therapy for MM patients who have average resources, the following can be done:

- Choose moderate forms of treatment, e.g. targeted therapies.
- Aim for the chronic illness scenario, i.e. don't aim for cure but for quality of life.
- Participate in clinical trials to extend resources.

There is much hope for patients whose treatments are individualized to suit themselves; their family members and friends; their tolerance of side effects, their will and motivation to be cured; and the resources that they possess. The key is finding the right balance that works.

Chapter **6**

MULTIPLE MYELOMA

"Step back and take a good look around; it's only logical that MM behaves like this."

Multiple Myeloma

This is the most important section in this book. In an effort to emphasize that some form of paradigm shift is desperately needed for us to provide better care and hope for patients with MM, I have decided to do this somewhat cross-grain. Instead of writing a regular literature review on established concepts, I would prefer to delve on fresher and newer concepts of disease biology and therapeutic targeting. I believe that only by challenging the conventional will we ever move forward in the way we approach and treat patients with MM or whatever disease. Literature reviews have been more expertly done by numerous and considerably more pre-eminent authors than I in the past. In all honesty, I have very little to add to those gems. But under some of those rocks, lie even greater treasures. Patients stand to gain much more from their doctors if we help them look under the rocks for new information; and this is exactly what I intend to do. In reality, all the medical literature that is available publicly is only the tip of the iceberg of the amount of knowledge that is present or will eventually be known.

Even at this very moment, there is much unpublished medical literature that for whatever reason would never ever get written or read. Obviously, it is not going to be possible in this book to tell you what lies beneath every rock, and it is certainly not my intention to do so. Instead, I would like to show you what lies beneath the rocks in my collection. I will present a large part of my own lesser published data to hopefully tell a "new" and logical story about this rather bewildering disease. Moreover, I hope to demonstrate that by applying this knowledge using more logical reasoning, I have indeed improved the clinical outcome of patients without the need for too many fancy and/or devastating modalities of therapy. The finesse to this is being able to achieve the desired results using regimens that are tailor-made to each individual. This will come with practice, lots of lots of logical reasoning, and a permissive environment.

I have always regarded broad concepts (rather than minutiae) as the key elements that will eventually guide therapy in all patients. Precise decimal-point dosing does not make any sense if you have used the wrong agent. We have all woken up in the morning with different moods. What's to stop a disease like MM to behave differently today as compared to yesterday? Are we so naïve to believe that 40 mg of dexamethasone today will give the same result as yesterday or tomorrow? Have we failed to realize that the problem is not just MM but the rest of the body? All of our bodies are made up of individual parts that are waking up differently every morning. Individualization requires us to cater to all these parts. This task is very frankly impossible. On the other hand, doing the opposite, i.e. having one size to fit all, is sweeping the dust under the carpet. The simplistic analogy for individualized therapy is really housekeeping. You'll have to do it daily and constantly. And everyone living in the house needs to put in his/her effort. The broad concepts are to identify key issues that need specific management — e.g. dust, trash, clothes, etc. Similarly, in MM, the broad concepts include the disease biology, the BM microenvironment, the blood supply and the immune system (Fig. 6.1). Don't miss the woods for the trees. There is a lot of information out there in today's high-tech

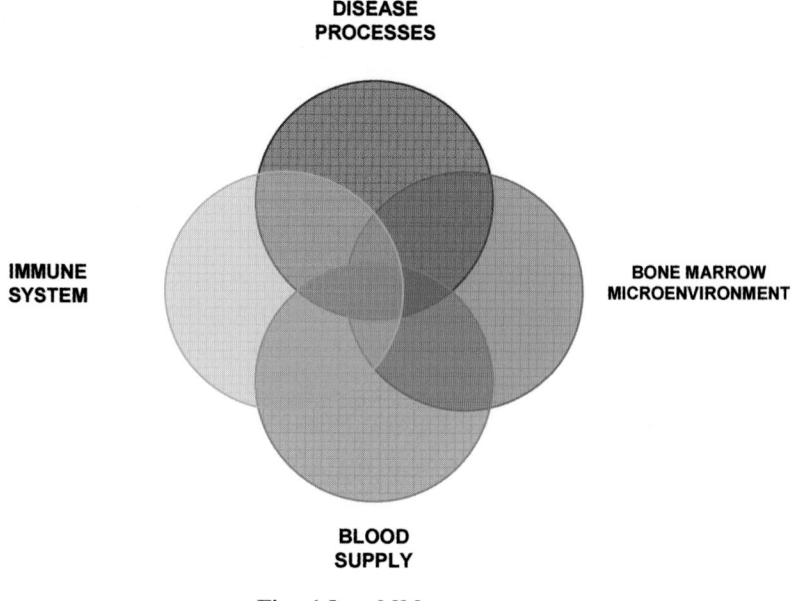

Fig. 6.1. MM parameters.

medical world; but very little of this is truly relevant. Data junk-yards are booming and bursting in concert with public and private affluence in the pursuit of cure, for example genomics and proteomics, i.e. the super high-definition studies of genes and proteins. Not that we should not pursue knowledge, but we are really spending more and getting less. Are we just like the music industry, where it's getting harder and harder to score a hit? Only a couple of decades ago, artistes like Sinatra, Elvis and the Fab Four churned out hit after hit, which we still listen to with pleasure. Today, however, the capacity to do this appears to have dwindled down. Every new song sounds like it was borrowed from an old one. We seem to have hit some level of finiteness. It's as though we cannot write a new tune anymore for humankind. Have we similarly hit some finiteness in the agents we have today?

The honest answer, fortunately, is that we clearly haven't. Today, the biotechnology and pharmaceutical industry, aided by a surge of highly-sophisticated technologies, have been bursting at the seams with new drugs and compounds. And the list grows almost daily.

So much so that we have created a unique problem, as a result of our successes, when we are selecting treatment for patients. There is no lack of agents to treat MM; we just don't have the knowledge of how to more effectively use them. I would in fact state categorically that instead of finding more and more new agents, it is probably more worthwhile, cost-effective and beneficial to patients that we put in more effort to figure out how to better and more logically use these agents. If we in the healthcare industry are truly pursuing cures for our patients, we should be putting on our thinking caps and using our true creativity, rather than pursuing that rare "hole-in-one."

Hence, in this section of the book, I will attempt to demonstrate to you how we could be creative and "think-out-of-the-box," and logically select treatment that is individually suitable for different patients. This might seem unconventional to some but the exercise is one that is not to satisfy the astute scientist and physician, but to challenge conventional dogma for the betterment of treatment outcome in MM. To do this, I will deliberately write in a style that is readable to the layperson for precisely that reason, i.e. I am appealing to the man/woman-in-the-street to consider his/her options carefully and to make a learned choice on how he/she should decide on his/her treatment. The reader is of course free to critique, agree or disagree with my views. The proof of the pudding is in the eating — treating patients in this manner (i.e. individualizing treatment) has resulted in extraordinary results in a sizable fraction of more than a hundred patients that have been specifically studied in detail. I will do this discussion as a narrative of the journey in the development of a protocol called "dtZ," for dexamethasone, thalidomide and zoledronic acid.

If Only Time Travel Were Possible

I have the habit of reading the last chapter of the book first. That's because I hate to lose the meaning of the book. I also hate re-reading anything and/or getting confused with what I'd read. Reading the last chapter first also helps one decide quickly if the rest of the book is worth reading, and to ditch it for another as early as possible so that the enjoyment is uninterrupted. In a similar way, if you could look into the crystal ball and figure out what the end results of treatment were like, you could make better decisions on treatment. Knowing what's to be expected at the end of the tunnel is like seeing the light beyond the twists and turns. If I had a disease like MM, I'd sure want to know.

Because some therapies are potentially permanently harmful, looking into the crystal ball is not a bad idea at all. Therapies that are designed to harm and damage cancer cells (as well as normal "innocent bystander" tissue) in fact do just that permanently and such a risk should strongly be considered from the time the diagnosis is made, i.e. before treatment is even commenced. Hence, the true value of this book is to the patient who is naïve in any form of treatment, who wants to know what's to be expected and in store for him/her in his/her long journey towards "cure." If only time travel were possible, then this book would be entirely obsolete, since permanence and irreversibility would then be themselves obsolete. But until the time when time travel becomes possible, this book is your crystal ball.

The key sub-parameters that relate to the disease are:

- The cancerous processes that operate within the MM cell.
- The BM microenvironment.
- The blood supply.
- The immune system.

Disease Processes

Group Dynamics of Molecular Events

Let's begin by considering the biology of the MM cell and relating this to the development of MM. There are a gazillion possibilities when you consider how complex and ramifying these interactions are. I have narrowed the scope of these interactions down to six dimensions that interact dynamically as a group. These need to be considered (as a group) before one can make a clear judgment of that snapshot in time of the status of that patient's MM:

- Single molecules.
- Two molecules interacting in a molecular reaction.
- Third-party molecules that influence that molecular reaction.
- Time, which fundamentally determines which third-party molecules are permitted to interact at that snapshot in time.
- Treatments (drugs and compounds) that influence the molecular interactions; they can potentially transect the effects that are being mediated by time.
- The summary of these events that are permutated because the affect similar downstream interactions.

The basic concepts of molecular interactions are shown in Fig. 6.2. Let's presume that there are two molecules (usually proteins) that interact abnormally in cancer cells, Molecules 1A and 2A (Fig. 6.2A). The products of this interaction are usually two modified molecules, Molecules 1B and 2B. Third-party molecules, e.g. Third-Party Molecule 1, may influence this reaction by, e.g. changing the speed of the reaction (Fig. 6.2B). This could in turn change the biological function in the MM cell, e.g. prevent DNA repair, and lead to serious consequences. If several of these third-party molecules (e.g. Third-Party Molecules 2 and 3) act on the same reaction (Fig. 6.2C), then the outcome can be very different. If in addition, these events are constantly changing in time and/or are influenced by drugs and treatments (Fig. 6.2D), then numerous permutations may occur at the same point of an otherwise relatively simple molecular reaction. The point to appreciate is that this is just one of the thousands of reactions that are occurring in the cancer cell. Moreover, reactions also occur between cancer proteins and normal/other cancer proteins. And third-party proteins can first affect other third-party proteins before affecting the main reaction. And so on and so forth. This means that understanding the context in which cancer cells operate are just as

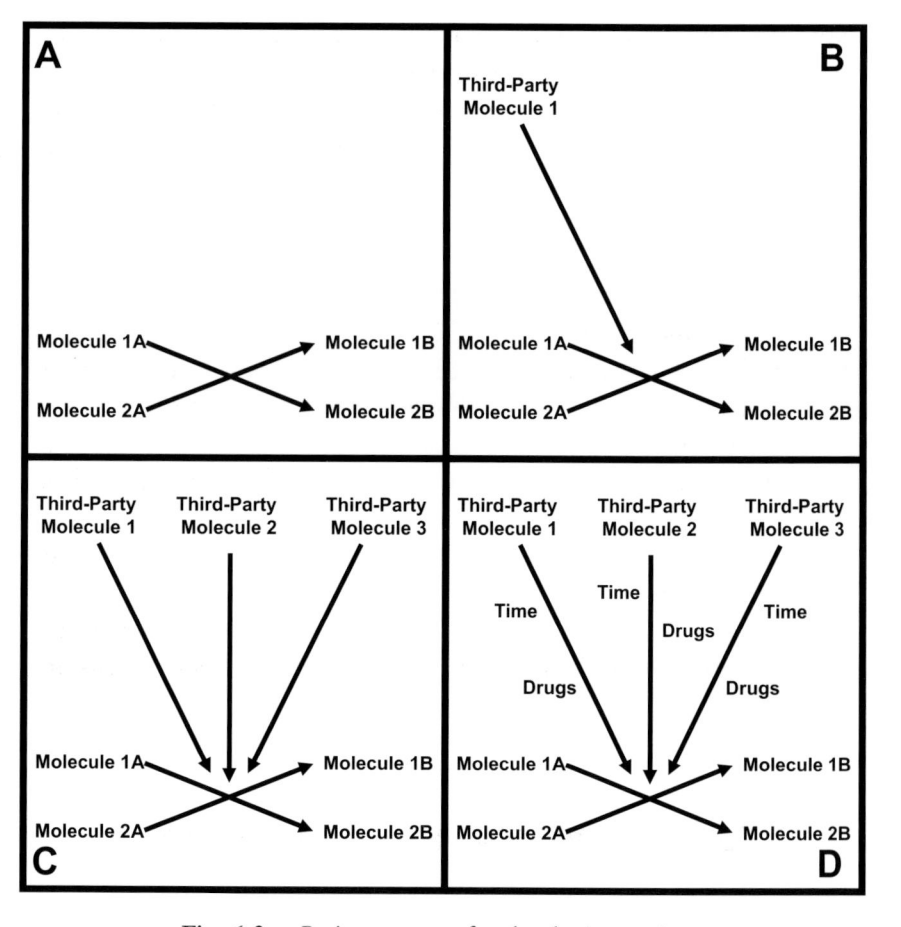

Fig. 6.2. Basic concepts of molecular interactions.

critical as knowing what the molecules are when we are selecting treatment for our patients. For example, abnormal proteins that are involved in red cell production might have no contextual relevance when the hemoglobin is normal, as when the hemoglobin is very low.

The Nature of Cancer Proteins

All proteins are composed of regions, domains or motifs. Most of these motifs accord some function to the cancer protein; and some are very much functionless. For example, protein domains may include DNA-binding domains, or regions of the protein that are more susceptible to digestion by other proteins (e.g. by the enzymes papain or pepsin). There are still other parts of a protein that can bind to other proteins and molecules in a lock-and-key fashion with extreme specificity. Other parts of the same protein may influence other cellular functions, e.g. growth stimulation. For the purposes of this book, it is not important to know what all these domains can do. Rather, it is more important to know that cancer proteins can be shorter, longer, same length, swapped around, duplicated, and modified in almost any way (Fig. 6.3). When such modifications occur, normal functions can be lost, and/or novel biological functions can arise. Upstream domains can even affect downstream functions. Domains that render the protein vulnerable to degradation, whether by other proteins or spontaneously, may greatly influence function as the half-life of such proteins will be very much shortened.

So how does knowing this help us decide on therapy? The principal consideration is the inherent instability that cancer cells harbor,

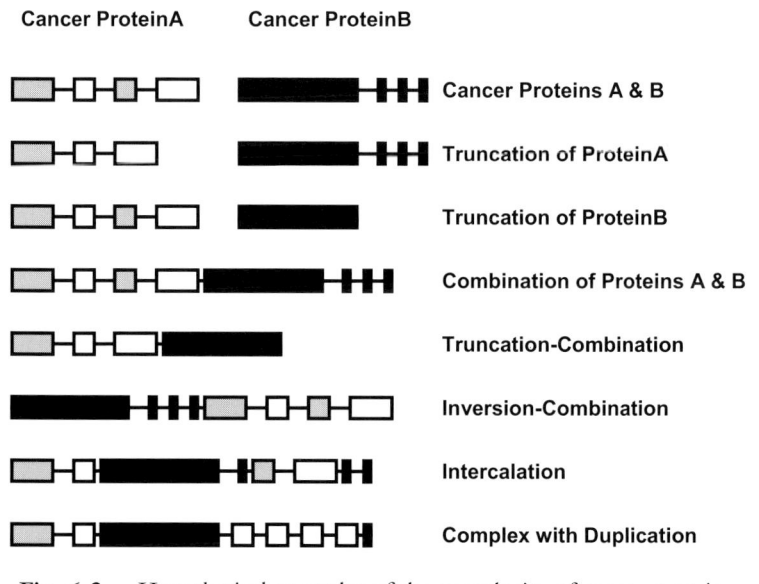

Fig. 6.3. Hypothetical examples of the complexity of cancer proteins.

out of sight and right under our noses. The important point is for us to recognize that things might not be like what they seem; that the books and papers might not be able to prepare us fully for the unexpected. If we go away thinking that one person's lung cancer is the same as another and that you can simply whip out that cancer treatment cookbook and apply your favorite regimen with equal success, you have failed immediately to appreciate that cancer cells (including MM cells) do not follow the ground rules. The point that I want to emphasize is awareness. Awareness that the unexpected is going to happen and that the explanation of why it happened might be overwhelmingly difficult. From a practical point of view, it is probably way too difficult in this day and age to pinpoint precisely the problem. Perhaps in the future all this might be possible. Accordingly, I, or for that matter any other doctor, might not have any answers for the patient in this situation. The best recourse could be to change to something totally different, since what has been tried is clearly not working.

More About Cancer Proteins

In trying to understand cancer proteins better, researchers have categorized them into two varieties: (i) loss of function (LOF) proteins and (ii) gain of function (GOF) proteins. Proteins are the functional units of life. Without proteins, there is basically no life. The codes for making proteins are contained in the many strands of DNA in each cell but DNA itself has no direct biological function. All of the cell's biological processes are dependent on proteins. This is the logical argument. A cancerous cell only behaves cancerous because some alteration in protein function gives it advantages for survival and growth (or proliferation). The effect is the failure of programmed cell death (or apoptosis[19]) and cell longevity. Even if there are changes in the DNA sequence that do not bring about a change in protein function, the cell will behave like a normal cell. Only when protein function has been altered will the cell behave as a cancer cell. If the normal biological process of a particular protein in the cell is one that leads to apoptosis, then a loss of that function in that protein could lead to cancer. In that scenario, the protein is now a cancer protein (or oncoprotein) due to a loss of function (LOF). In contrast, if that protein has changed such that it now is able to promote growth of the cell, resulting in cancer, then the protein is called a gain of function (GOF) oncoprotein.

Here is the convoluted line of thought. I must ask that you first free your mind from the normal perception of what cancer is and consider the following slowly and sequentially. Whether LOF or GOF, let's first say that a certain oncoprotein is able to confer an advantage to the cell over other cells. Neither survival nor proliferative advantage actually makes this cell a cancer cell until the effects are clearly malicious. For example, burst growth of white blood cells in response to an infection by bacteria is not considered malicious but is appropriate, protective and reparative. Even when burst growth of white blood cells of a catastrophic nature occurs in response to a germ (pathogen, e.g. severe acute respiratory syndrome, SARS, virus), which eventually leads to the death of the patient, the disease is not considered a cancer. In other words, a survival and/or growth advantage accorded to a cell which leads to a disease that can be fatal is not necessarily a cancer. Yet even when there is an increase in the proteins of the cells that mediate survival and growth biological pathways, this is insufficient to call this disease a cancer, as even normal cells in burst growth can demonstrate increases in cell survival and growth proteins. What then is a cancer?

Now the lines start to gray out and get fuzzy. They get even fuzzier when some cancers, e.g. liver cancer and cervical cancer, are known to be caused by viral infections, e.g. hepatitis B virus (HBV) and human papillomavirus (HPV), respectively. Moreover, we can prevent the respective cancers from developing by immunizing ourselves against HBV and HPV. In other words, we can prevent cancer by preventing infection. So then can SARS be considered an explosive cancer? Well, certainly SARS is associated with other features of cancer like spreading ("metastasis") to other organs and reliance on growth factors (or cytokines). But SARS is not a cancer. Growth and survival advantages of cells that are mediated by (i) changes in LOF and GOF proteins; (ii) metastases; (iii) cytokine-mediated growth; and (iv) increases in proteins that mediate cell survival and cell growth are all not sufficient to reach a diagnosis of cancer.

Cancer has two major hallmarks that distinguish it from other diseases — clonality and maliciousness. Clonality means that the cancer cells are uniformly distinguishable as identical copies of each other. Clonality implies that there is a central ("mother") cell (or cancer stem cell) that is responsible for producing these cell copies (or clones). Consequently, these clonal cells are conferred a greater capacity of survival and growth which they engage with a fervor to the point of "bullying" other cells and tissues around them (see below in the sections on the BM microenvironment and blood supply). Their maliciousness in disregarding the normally harmonious cell-to-cell interactions in the body permits them to gain territory and the necessary supplies for their "selfish" needs. Moreover, the lack of orderly regulation progresses to frank aggression against the normal surveillance processes that ensure peace and harmony in the body, i.e. the immune system. Cancer not only attacks the immune system, cancer will coerce and even con the immune system for its own advantage. With the immune system blind to it, cancer cells now expand and extend to all parts of the body, setting up satellites (or metastases) in tissues far remote from its original home. Its fearless greed eventually turns against itself. The whole body is now totally ravaged by this monster, which has been called the "crab" (cancer is the Latin word for crab), and becomes emancipated. Yet the disease gives no signs that it will even decelerate or let alone stop; and death ensues. Indeed, and almost cliché, only till death will cancer part.

The Relationship of Gene Abnormalities to Cancer

Genetic abnormalities that are present in cancer cells do not define these cells as cancer cells. Cancer cells with a completely normal genetic repertoire can behave like cancer cells. Such is the paradox in MM, where MM cells that are genetically normal might even be more aggressive than MM cells that contain genetic abnormalities (e.g. having more than the usual number of strands of DNA/chromosomes, called hyperdiploidy). Whilst some genetic abnormalities confer survival and growth advantages to the cancer cell, it is equally conceivable that other abnormalities might indeed confer disadvantages. Hence, a balance of sorts is met when the ying and the yang have exerted their respective influences. (I will return to the discussion on the relevance of genetic abnormalities in cancer a little later in the book.)

So, regardless of the genetic environment that cancer cells flourish in, there has to be some disorder in the regulation (dysregulation) of the biological processes of survival and/or growth of that cell in order for it to express the biological behavior of cancerous cells. In addition, this has to occur in all the cellular copies of that clone. By logical reasoning, there then has to be at least one oncoprotein responsible for that dysregulation, since the biological function of a cancer cell is after all performed by proteins and not by genes. I agree that abnormal cancer genes (or oncogenes) that produce abnormal oncoproteins might lead to a cell behaving in a cancerous way. I however argue that normal genes can also eventually produce abnormal proteins that could behave the same way as oncoproteins, and lead to the development of cancer. I further challenge age-old rhetoric and state categorically that gene signatures that are found in cancer cells might even be secondary effects of an ongoing cancerous process and are not the origin of a cancer at all. The analogy is of course the red herring.

In reality, there are probably numerous oncoproteins interacting in coordinated and uncoordinated biological pathways. Today, using the laboratory tools that we have, probably only the tip of the iceberg of these pathways have been detected. Some of these are directly driven by oncogenes, whilst others are driven by disorderly biological processes in the cells that deal with the way abnormal proteins are degraded by a cell's built-in garbage disposal system. Remarkably, in some situations, nothing abnormal can be detected. That we do not detect any oncoproteins really doesn't mean that there aren't any; we just couldn't detect them with our methods and skills. We have simply reached the limits of scientific knowledge. Indeed, cancer cells are sometimes holed up in a secret part

84 *Towards Individualized Therapy for Multiple Myeloma*

of the body and are extremely difficult to find — almost akin to what a terrorist might do. Accordingly, if the doctor tells a patient that nothing abnormal has been found (i.e. oncoprotein or oncogene), this does not exclude the presence of cancer or discount the malicious effects of the disease.

The Biology of MM in a Different Light

If you refer to the journals, internet or bookstores, you will find loads and loads of writings on MM — from its origin to its termination. If you read these articles, very soon you will find that you are reading the same thing again and again. In other words, there is only so much that we know of MM and every other MM investigator or advocate is trying to say it in a "different" way hoping that by doing that it would be sufficiently novel for publication and reading. Worse still, we also find reprints and re-editions of the same article giving us the same information. For the patient, this is indeed bad news because with so much invested in research, all we have is the same old rhetoric. We desperately need to see it in a different light.

As I have discussed above, oncoproteins are a prerequisite for cells to behave like cancer cells. In stripping MM down to its bare bones, it is well-known that even an entirely normal genetic makeup can be found in MM cells. And this is happening in the face of ultra-sophisticated genetic/genomic testing, where no gene is excluded from scrutiny. This seemingly basic observation is extremely critical because it strongly challenges the genetic theory of cancer and MM. In addition, even if gene abnormalities were found, they would not be capable of telling us whether these lead to the development of MM because they are like snapshots in time. In other words, such genetic abnormalities (if found) could well be secondary events that arose after transformation to cancer had already occurred, and not the transformational events themselves. A cause and effect relationship cannot be ascribed even if gene abnormalities were found. Unfortunately, protein science lags far behind genetics/genomics. Gene arrays are far easier to perform

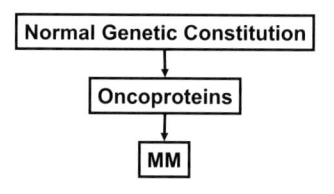

Fig. 6.4. Bare bones about MM.

and analyze than protein arrays. And even if we find the proteins from protein arrays, again, as a snapshot in time, we might not be able to say if they were the primary maligners. But returning to the basic schema in Fig. 6.4, it is easy to draw logic on how maliciousness can operate in an MM cell, but the second issue of clonality may be much more difficult to fit in. Certainly normal cells with normal genetic constitutions are not considered clones, or else we would all be clonal. Yet MM cells with normal genetic makeup can behave as clones. Does clonality occur before oncoproteins are formed or after or together?

In the model of clonality that I would like to propose, let us assume that oncoproteins are formed *de novo* and they confer survival and growth advantages to the cell. In other words, oncoproteins that are formed by whatever mechanism can potentially lead to cell transformation (into cancer). Cellular transformation would permit that cell to expand itself over and above all other cells until clonality is achieved (Fig. 6.5). If this cell is already capable of burst proliferation when in its untransformed state, then it is possible

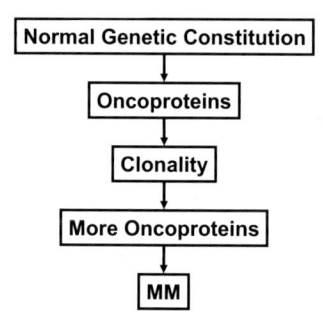

Fig. 6.5. MM clonality.

86   *Towards Individualized Therapy for Multiple Myeloma*

that when these signals are encountered after transformation, it will undergo rapid clonal expansion as well. After attaining clonality, cancer cells can continue in their expansion towards being a tumor as well as spread to other satellite sites via the original oncoproteins or newer ones. This model in fact fits very nicely for MM principally because the normal counterparts of MM cells are the plasma cells, which during a normal immunological event called B lymphocyte (or B cell) maturation, are fully capable of burst proliferation. In fact, the capacity of explosive growth in normal B cells is the highest amongst all cell types.

Universal Hallmark of MM — Isotype Class Switch Recombination (iCSR)

More than 10 years ago, Professor Kenneth Anderson and I reviewed numerous scientific papers that were available at that time and came to a conclusion that the single most important hallmark of MM was iCSR.[20] This process, iCSR, is a feature of normal B cells and plasma cells. It involves a genetic event in the IgH gene that is located in the long arm of chromosome number 14. The precise gene location for the more scientifically-minded amongst us is chromosome 14q32 ("q" for the long arm of chromosome 14; and "32" for gene locus position 32 on that arm). Other researchers at that time had also found that nearly all patients with MM had genetic abnormalities at the chromosome 14q32 locus and suggested that these genetic events were virtually universal for MM.[21] Amongst all the laboratory data for MM, this finding has been the most intriguing to me because burst proliferation of normal B cells must involve molecular pathways that affect chromosome 14q32. It is not difficult to then assume that MM cells would also undergo burst proliferation when given the same signals that would induce their normal B cell counterparts to proliferate rapidly.

In normal iCSR that occurs in normal B cells, the class of Ig switches from a less mature one to a more mature one. Specifically, IgM switches over to IgG or IgA or IgE. (There is another Ig called IgD that is secreted in very minute quantities which I will ignore for the purposes of this discussion.) For all intents and purposes, in relation to MM, we only observe the clones of IgG or IgA or IgE, and not IgM. Patients who have clonal production of IgM have a related condition called Waldenstrom's macroglobulinemia, which behaves differently from MM. I will also deliberately exclude Waldenstrom's macroglobulinemia from this discussion so that I will not confuse readers further. The point to emphasize is that in the development (or pathogenesis, or myelomagenesis) of MM, there is a distinct event that is observed that heralds the onset of MM, i.e. iCSR. Pre-cancerous (or pre-malignant, or precursor) MM cells are thought to be IgM-secreting B (or plasma) cells, which are also known as memory B cells. Upon undergoing iCSR and transformation, these IgM B cells become IgG or IgA or IgE and take on the cancerous characteristics of MM. Because burst proliferation is built into iCSR by nature, this transforming event also accelerates the expansion of clonal malignant plasma cells. So to summarize the impact of iCSR on myelomagenesis:

- iCSR is a biological process in normal B or plasma cells.
- iCSR involves genetic changes in the IgH gene at the gene locus 14q32.
- Before iCSR, normal B or plasma cells, as well as pre-malignant precursor MM cells are IgM-secreting cells.
- After iCSR, Ig secretion becomes IgG or IgA or IgE depending on how Ig class switching has occurred.
- MM cells are frequently IgG or IgA or IgE, but almost never IgM. In addition, abnormalities of the IgH 14q32 gene locus are observed in virtually all patients with MM. Collective these data suggest that iCSR is a universal hallmark of MM.
- Because iCSR is potentially transforming and associated with rapid burst proliferation of plasma cells, abnormalities occurring during iCSR could result in myelomagenesis and clonal expansion of malignant plasma cells.

Unfortunately, we do not have direct evidence today that any of this is true. However, it continues to remain to be one of the

88   *Towards Individualized Therapy for Multiple Myeloma*

hypotheses of the origin of MM which I embrace and is the subject of continued research and investigations.

More Intriguing Data on iCSR and Myelomagenesis

In order for normal B cells to undergo iCSR, a peculiar and rather major genetic event must occur. This is called DNA double-strand break repair (DSBR). DNA as you know is basically a very, very long chain of sugar molecules wound around like a long ribbon. It is remarkably stable and can be extracted even from dead cells after several years. With the laboratory tools we have today, one could even purify DNA, dry it in a tiny bottle, ship it by snail mail across the world, reconstitute at its final destination, insert it into living cell (e.g. bacteria) and observe its functions with 100% fidelity. In iCSR, the cell needs to break up this double-stranded DNA ribbon, remove the unwanted segments and repair everything with 100% fidelity. The difference is that the patient actually has absolutely no control over how it happens and anything can go wrong. In fact, this phenomenon is known as genomic instability and nature has built this tendency to mutate at the 14q32 gene locus into all B cells to permit them to function and protect us from foreign invaders, e.g. bacteria and viruses. Genomic instability is not a regular feature of all cells. If it were, all cells would mutate at will and there would be absolute mayhem. Genomic instability is provided by nature to a select group of cells in the immune system to permit sufficient flexibility for it to cope with foreign insults. It is my hypothesis that in MM, this process has gone awfully wrong.

In all normal cells, and not just B cells or plasma cells, a number of enzymes are involved in DSBR. One of the most important of these is DNA protein kinase (DNA-PK). This enzyme is considered a giant amongst enzymes and proteins, weighing in at more than 200 kilo Daltons (kDa). It is composed of two sections: (i) a part that does the DSBR function, called the catalytic subunit (CS); and another part that regulates the repair function of CS, called the regulatory subunit. The regulatory subunit is made up to two proteins called Ku70 and Ku86. Hence, DNA-PK is also known as DNA-PK$_{CS}$-Ku70-Ku86. Again, as expected, DNA-PK is found inside the nucleus of the cell where the DNA is. When the cell encounters an insult that damages the DNA strand, e.g. X-rays, that cell needs to repair the DNA break. If the DNA is only partially broken (i.e. one of the two strands is broken), then DNA repair is relatively easy to perform using the other strand as a template; like filling in the blank pieces of a nearly completed jigsaw puzzle. This is called homologous recombination (HR). However, when both strands of the DNA ribbon are broken, the problem is escalated by volumes. There are freely hanging ends of broken DNA that must now find each other in the dark, and then get filled in or reconnected in the appropriate manner. This process of DNA repair is known as DSBR by non-homologous end joining (NHEJ).

What if there are many broken parts because of more extensive DNA damage? Then the appropriate DNA partner ends might not meet and join up with the appropriate partners. Accordingly, these loose DNA ends must find "consenting" partners to join with. These alliances have been curiously and rather aptly termed "promiscuous" chromosomal translocations. In the case of MM, the DNA double-strand break occurs at the IgH 14q32 gene locus as part of the iCSR event. However, there could be other DNA double-strand breaks in the rest of the genome occurring simultaneously. During DSBR by NHEJ, these other DNA ends could be translocated to the IgH 14q32 gene locus and lead to a chromosomal translocation. Because studies in numerous patients with MM have shown that the IgH 14q32 gene locus associates itself with a huge variety of "consenting" translocation partners, it is considered a highly promiscuous locus. Hence, it is precisely these promiscuous chromosomal translocations that occur at the IgH 14q32 gene locus that are the hallmark of MM. Let me summarize again:

- In iCSR, the target gene locus is IgH 14q32.
- The process involves DSBR by NHEJ.
- Because random DNA double-strand breaks might also occur in the rest of the genome and NHEJ is a risky process.

90   *Towards Individualized Therapy for Multiple Myeloma*

- A large variety of "consenting" chromosomal partners converge at the IgH 14q32 gene locus.
- Thus the chromosomal translocations occurring at IgH 14q32 are not only universal; they are highly promiscuous; and this is the universal hallmark of MM.

The Turning Point — CD40

The evidence above suggests that DSBR in MM has gone awfully wrong. Yet, there was no clue at that time as to what could have gone wrong. Like all things in science, it was serendipity that led Professor Kenneth Anderson (Ken), I and my team of researchers to uncover some of this mystery. The work started back in 1995 when I was at the Dana-Farber Cancer Institute (DFCI) in Boston. Ken had just obtained a new molecule that triggers a cell membrane receptor called the CD40 receptor.[22] This triggering molecule was very simply called CD40 ligand (CD40L). There is a disease, called the X-Linked Hyperimmunoglobulin M (HyperIgM) Syndrome, where patients are unable to produce IgG or IgA or IgE, but are only able to produce IgM. In other words, patients with X-Linked HyperIgM Syndrome have a problem with iCSR. These patients actually suffer from serious immune deficiency (or immunodeficiency) and are lacking CD40L. Since the gene for CD40L resides in the X chromosome, only male members of the family suffer from this condition because males have only one X chromosome. As expected, normal B cells and plasma cells express the CD40 receptor on their cell membranes. In fact, most MM cells also do. So, Ken wanted to examine what would happen to the MM cell if CD40 was triggered. However, unlike normal B cells and plasma cells where a second signal (i.e. interleukin-4, IL-4) was required to trigger complete iCSR (Fig. 6.6A), this second signal (IL-4) was not provided (Fig. 6.6B) in the experiments that I will describe below.

As mentioned above, normal iCSR requires CD40L and IL-4 as co-triggering molecules to complete iCSR (Fig. 6.6A). In the above

A – Normal B Cell iCSR

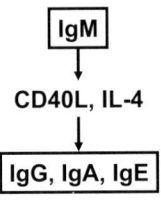

B – CD40L Experiment on MM Cells

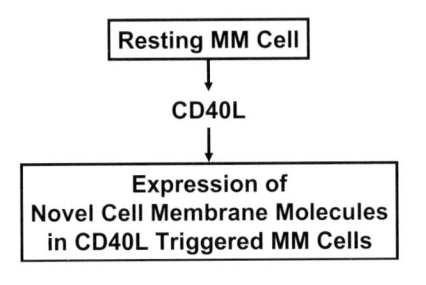

Fig. 6.6. CD40 and IL-4 triggering in iCSR.

experiment (Fig. 6.6B), only CD40L is provided as a pure trigger for MM cells. And the aim of the experiment was to see if there are any novel molecules on the cell membrane of MM cells that could be uncovered by the CD40L signal. It was an interesting hypothesis because the expectation was zero, since iCSR was a cellular event that occurred in the nucleus and not the cell surface, and only half the signal was provided, albeit trying to make the experiment as pure as possible. The results however were pivotal in that it completely changed the way I approached MM.

CD40L Induces Burst Proliferation of MM Cells

The first observation was not entirely surprising: CD40L induced burst proliferation of MM cells. However, this did not occur in normal B cells.[23] Normal B cells require both signals, CD40L as well as IL-4. There was for the first time something abnormal in the biological processes (not the end result) of iCSR in MM cells that we could detect. This finding greatly influenced the subsequent experiments that followed. Permit me to just summarize the data before we proceed further:

At a very superficial level, the least one can conclude is that MM cells behave differently from normal B cells (Table 6.1). At the minimum, IL-4 signaling is decoupled from CD40L in MM cells. Perhaps MM cells have their own way of making IL-4 or triggering the IL-4 receptor without the need for more IL-4. The logical conclusion is that this is not unexpected since one is a normal cell and the other a cancerous cell, so there must be some detectable difference. The point here is not so much what was observed, but that there was now a tool to separate the two, a chance to find out why the MM cell is a cancer. And the "umph" of this finding is that the triggering molecule is right at the heart of MM itself, a direct link to the universal hallmark of MM, iCSR. Many researchers, I bet, will home in next on IL-4 signaling cascades in MM. But here lies the finesse; we chose to put our last dollar on CD40L instead. Incidentally and just for the record, round about that time many researchers were working on a cousin of IL-4, i.e. IL-6, which was then found to be the most important exogenous growth factor for MM. So whilst most were triggering MM cells using IL-6 and working out the survival and growth pathways downstream of the iCSR event, we were working at the heart of iCSR.

Table 6.1. CD40L and/or IL-4 Triggering of MM Cells and Normal B Cells and Cell Proliferation

Trigger	MM Cells	Normal B Cells
CD40L	Burst proliferation	No change
IL-4	No change	No change
CD40L & IL-4	No change	Burst proliferation

CD40L and Ku86

Over the next 8 to 10 years of experimentation, the triggering of MM cells using CD40L became progressively easier as cell-based assays gave way to recombinant human CD40L which was produced by fermentation in bacterial cells. This led to an exponential rise in our understanding of the biology which was at the heart of MM. In fact, the very next experiment provided a truly out-of-the-box concept that is intriguing me, even till today. As mentioned, we triggered both normal B cells as well as MM cells using CD40L and then injected these cells into separate experimental mice to see how the mice would react in an immunologically manner. The hope was to be able to detect in the mice anti-human antibodies (MAHA) that were specific for MM cells and not normal B cells. This would pave the way for us to perhaps detect, isolate and purify MM-specific tumor proteins (also called tumor-specific antigens, TSAs) that can be used to develop novel treatment strategies. Most interestingly, the very first MAHA we developed detected the Ku86 DNA repair protein. If you recall, Ku86 is one of the two units of the regulatory subunit of the DNA-PK_{CS}-Ku70-Ku86 repair enzyme that is involved in DSBR by NHEJ during iCSR. Needless to say, I fell off my chair when the results of the protein analysis were handed to us.

Because we were using whole cells rather than minced cells to inject the mice, the molecules that we were detecting were more likely cell membrane molecules, and not molecules that were within the cells. If that were the case, then finding Ku86 would imply that this molecule was expressed on the cell membrane, rather than in the nucleus of the cell where DNA repair would be expected to be occurring. In other words, Ku86 was not in its usual location. Indeed, we subsequently confirmed that Ku86 was located on the cell membrane of MM cells following CD40L triggering but far less frequently in non-triggered MM cells. I remember talking about this to many people in the research field and the summary of their responses is as follows:

- A very interesting observation with little or no value.
- Another very interesting observation with little or no value.
- Definitely a very interesting observation with little or no value.

94   *Towards Individualized Therapy for Multiple Myeloma*

At this point of time, one could do a few things, including: (i) throwing in the towel; (ii) doing a bungee jump and hoping that the strings snapped; or (iii) looking for another disease to treat. Fortunately, the Journal of Clinical Investigations (JCI) loved the idea and even gave us the cover. Then, another researcher reported something even more extraordinary that made me throw away my towel, my bungee ticket and my other textbook to continue pursuing CD40L and Ku86 in MM. A Japanese researcher (T. Morio) had found that Ku70 and Ku86 proteins were bound to the CD40 receptor on the surface of normal B cells when the cells were triggered using the physiological dual signals of CD40L and IL-4; and that they could be shuttled between the nucleus and the cell membrane.[24] This was simply amazing.

We of course wanted to know if this association was also observed in MM cells and performed an analysis called laser scanning confocal microscopy. As can be seen in Fig. 6.7 below, the MM cell indeed shows co-localization (yellow) of CD40 receptors (red) and Ku86 proteins (green). These were found both in the cytoplasm as well as the cell membrane. I would like to add that these observations were only seen in MM cells that were treated with the single signal

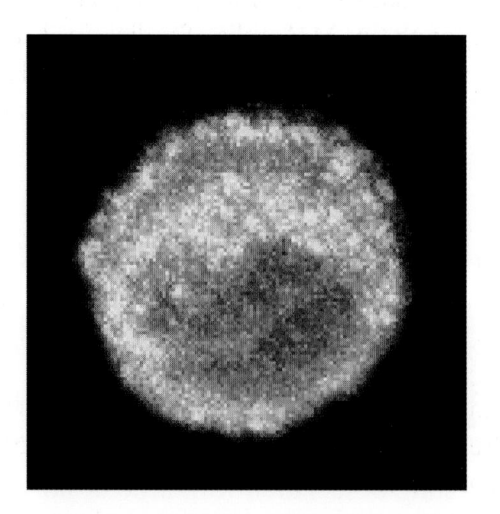

Fig. 6.7. Co-localization of CD40 and Ku86 on the cell membrane of MM cells.

Table 6.2. CD40L and/or IL-4 Triggering of MM Cells and Normal B Cells and CD40-Ku86 Co-Localization

Trigger	MM Cells	Normal B Cells
CD40L	CD40-Ku86 co-localization	No co-localization
IL-4	No co-localization	No co-localization
CD40L & IL-4	No co-localization	CD40-Ku86 co-localization

CD40L and not in the non-triggered cells, or MM cells triggered with either IL-4 alone or CD40L and IL-4. Although CD40L and Ku86 were similarly co-localized in both normal B cells as well as MM cells, the triggering signals required were different, i.e. CD40L and IL-4 in normal B cells and CD40L alone in MM cells (Table 6.2).

Variants of Ku86 Protein in MM Cells

The abnormal biology of Ku86 in MM cells provoked my research team to delve deeper into the significance of Ku86 in iCSR, the development of mutations (or mutagenesis), and the regulation of survival and growth in MM cells. Studies in Ku70 and Ku86 knockout mice (i.e. mice in which the Ku70 or Ku86 gene has been removed) have demonstrated both tumor suppressor (i.e. prevention of cancer formation) function as well as effects on the cell cycle and cell proliferation. These data suggest that there could be losses or gains of function for Ku70 and/or Ku86 proteins, i.e. just like oncoproteins. Hence, we hypothesized that Ku86 in MM could potentially be an oncoprotein for the following reasons:

- That variants of Ku86 protein have been reported in 86% to 100% of freshly isolated MM cells from MM patients.[25–27]
- That variants of Ku86 protein could associate with members of the apoptosis: antiapoptosis group of proteins (e.g. BAX and Bcl2).

96   *Towards Individualized Therapy for Multiple Myeloma*

Table 6.3.   Characteristics of Ku86 Variants in MM cells

Characteristics	Ku86v-N	Ku86v-C
Deletion	Rightward or C-Terminus	Leftward or N-Terminus
Molecule	N-Terminus	C-Terminus
Estimated Size	69 kDa	56 kDa
Functional Domain	Lost (LOF)	Preserved (GOF)
Nuclear Localization Signal (NLS)	Preserved	Deleted
Subcellular Location	Nucleus	Cytoplasm, cell membrane
Response to CD40L	Transport into the nucleus	Persistently attached to CD40 in the membrane
Principal Molecular Association	DNA-PK$_{CS}$	Bcl2
Impact on Function	Poor DNA repair	Potential oncoprotein

- That variants of Ku86 protein could associate with cell cycle regulatory proteins (e.g. CDK4 and E2F-4).

It is not possible to discuss the details of the subsequent studies without going into technical jargon, which will certainly leave the layman totally lost. Accordingly, I would prefer to stop by summarizing the findings on Ku86 variant proteins (Ku86v) in Table 6.3 above. Essentially, we performed a long string of experiments, including purifying Ku86v-C oncoprotein from the cell membrane; showing its association to the anti-apoptotic (cell survival and longevity) protein, Bcl2 in a 2-dimensional pull-down assay; and confirming its identity using mass spectrometry. The final molecule is so complicated in its alteration that it resembles one of the bizarre hypothetical proteins presented in Fig. 6.3. In concluding this section, I would first like to mention that the role of Ku86v-C as a putative oncoprotein is not established but still under investigation. The native freshly-formed Ku86 molecule is highly susceptible to digestion by enzymes that are naturally present in the cell. This is called proteolytic cleavage. Some of these enzymes might occur during activation of the normal precursor B cell. This means that the natural process of precursor B cell maturation may hypothetically induce the formation of a malicious oncoprotein. I reiterate that much of this is currently theoretical and speculative, but it provokes us to consider that cancerous processes can in fact piggyback and use normal biological functions of the cell for its malignant purposes. This idea is not entirely new, since viruses (because they possess no cellular machinery to maintain biological processes) do exactly this in order to survive, replicate and spread. Using this argument, I consider it highly likely that both Ku86v-N and Ku86v-C proteins are produced in this manner, perhaps through an external insult (e.g. ionizing radiation or X-rays) or through chance.

Proteins are actually like a string of beads with two free ends, called the amino- (N-) and carboxy- (C-) termini. In the Ku86 protein, the N-terminus contains a part of the protein that helps the protein enter the nucleus (i.e. a nuclear-localization signal or NLS); whereas the C-terminus contains the functional parts of the molecule, especially the DNA repair function. If the protein breakdown deletes most of the C-terminus, then the remaining shortened variant protein which retains the N-terminus (Ku86v-N) will lose its DNA repair function (Fig. 6.8). However, if the protein deletion is over at the other end, i.e. the N-terminus, then the remaining variant protein which retains the C-terminus (Ku-86v-C) would be expected to still keep its DNA repair function (Fig. 6.9). In other words, Ku86v-N is a LOF protein because of loss of DNA repair function (Fig. 6.8) and Ku86v-C is at least a functional molecule that is capable of repairing DNA breaks (Fig. 6.9). I will discuss why Ku86v-C could be a GOF protein later.

We and others had previously identified the LOF Ku86v-N protein and demonstrated the severely impaired DNA repair function. Even though Ku86v-N has kept its NLS and hence able to localize within the nucleus (where most of the DNA is usually found), it is unable to repair DNA because it lacks the enzyme functions contained in the C-terminus, since the C-terminus had been deleted. Experiments done on MM cells exposed to DNA damaging drugs, e.g. cytotoxic agents or chemotherapy drugs, have shown them to be unable to repair DNA and even die because of the cumulative

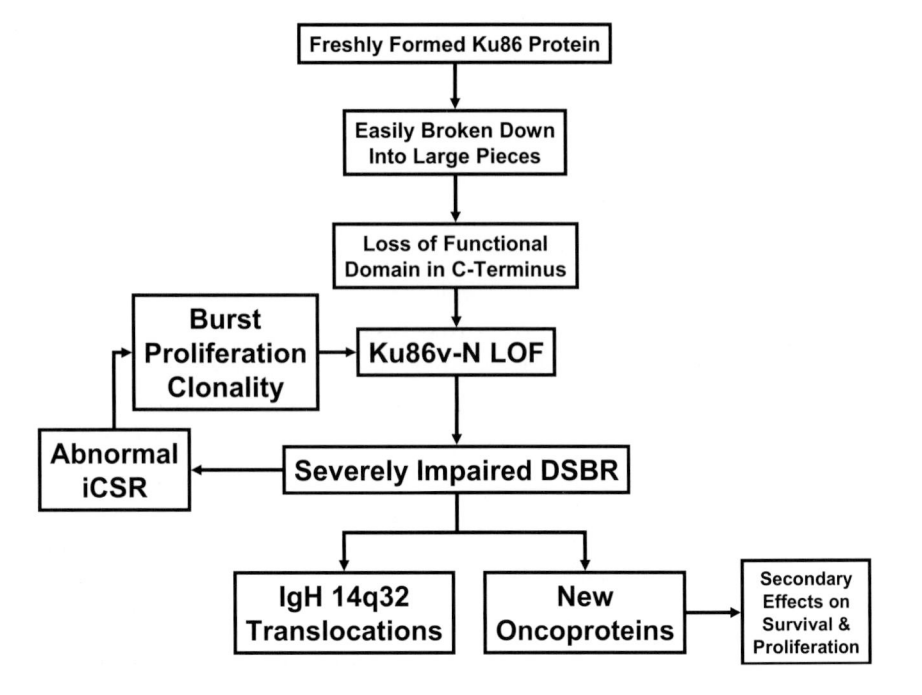

Fig. 6.8. Ku86v-N — loss of DNA repair function.

and severe DNA damage. This loss of DSBR could lead to abnormal iCSR and formation of an abnormal clone of MM cells, especially when under the influence of B cell activation signals (i.e. CD40L and/or IL-4). Indeed, as mentioned above, our studies have shown that the normal CD40L plus IL-4 signal is abnormal in MM cells[28] and specifically, that CD40L alone (i.e. without IL-4) is required for activation of MM cells that leads to burst proliferation of MM cells. Our studies have further demonstrated that CD40L very rapidly causes new genetic abnormalities in MM cells; suggesting that the CD40-triggered MM cell could undergo clonal evolution. We postulate the following:

• That the initial burst proliferation of a precursor MM cell that has become abnormal as a result of impaired DSBR and abnormal iCSR, lead to the establishment of a clone of malignant plasma cells and the development of MM.

Multiple Myeloma 99

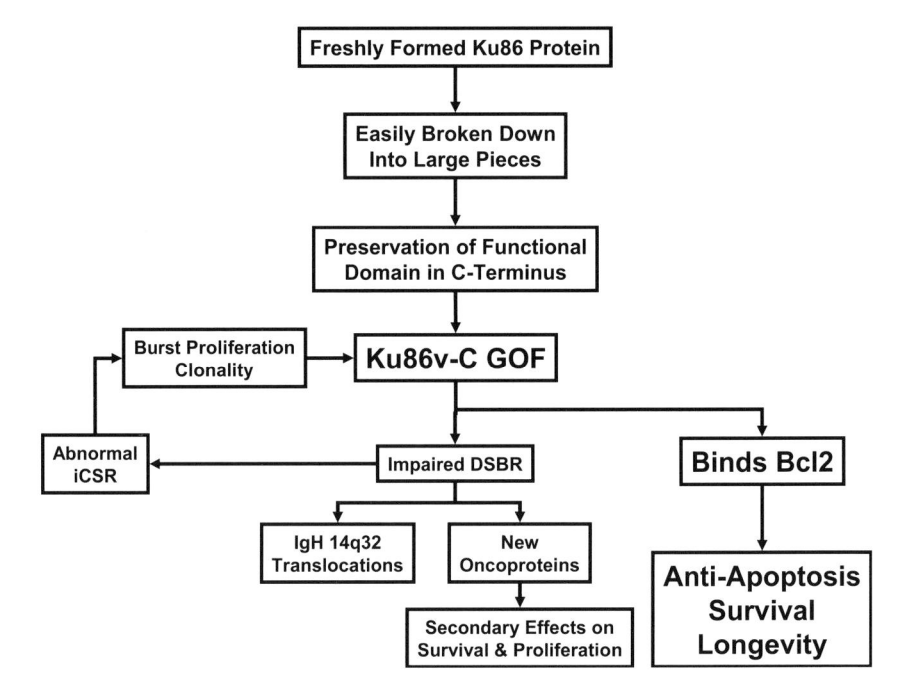

Fig. 6.9. Ku86v-C — putative oncoprotein.

- Severely impaired DSBR leading to IgH 14q32 translocations.
- Severely impaired DSBR could by chance lead to new onco-genes and oncoproteins that may impact on the survival and proliferation of MM cells.

The take home message for Ku86v-N is that it is the loss of DNA repair function that potentially causes problems typically seen in cancer cells, i.e. (i) resilience of clones of malignant cells, (ii) the presence of genetic abnormalities that progressively evolve, and (iii) the generation of potentially new oncoproteins. The situation is not the same for Ku86v-C (below), where there is potential for the variant Ku86v protein to be a true oncoprotein.

Let us assume that the variant Ku86v protein is formed by the same processes of protein digestion in the cell but this time the N-terminus is taken off. This leaves the C-terminus intact in the residual molecule. The loss of the N-terminus is associated with failure of the Ku86v-C protein (Fig. 6.9) to move into the nucleus to repair DNA, even though it possesses the functional parts of the protein that perform DNA repair in the C-terminus. This in fact leads to the same outcome as Ku86v-N, i.e. failure of DNA repair, but for a different reason. It is the inability of Ku86v-C to be contiguous with damaged DNA (and not the lack of function) that leads to impaired DSBR. In fact, we now find Ku86v-C in a new location, i.e. in the cell membrane, nearly outside the cell and well away from the nucleus. Interestingly, triggering MM cells via CD40 leads to yet greater accumulation of cell membrane Ku86 proteins, chiefly Ku86v-C, as well as the association of Ku86/Ku86v proteins with CD40 itself. The significance of this is at present unclear, but should Ku86/Ku86v proteins be able to trigger CD40, this could potentiate myelomagenic processes, i.e. biological processes that induce the development and progression of MM. Hence, via CD40 on the cell membrane, aberrantly located Ku86v-C protein could have an oncogenic role. Whereas, Ku86v-C protein has impaired DNA-repair function (i.e. LOF), this potentially oncogenic role could be considered as a gain of biological function.

Ku86 protein is well-known to bind to numerous proteins. We and others had previously investigated whether Ku86 binds to proteins that regulate the cell cycle, i.e. the cellular processes that cause a cell to grow and divide. Amongst the strongest associations of Ku86 were with cell cycle proteins called CDK4, E2F-4 and Bcl2. These cell cycle proteins regulate the cell cycle in a cascade fashion, where the cell signal is transferred from one protein to another. In general, there are two types of proteins, those that produce positive growth and/or survival effects, and those that produce negative effects. CDK4, E2F-4 and Bcl2 are all proteins that promote cell survival (anti-apoptosis) and/or proliferation. As mentioned above, one of the strongest associations of Ku86v is with the anti-apoptotic protein, Bcl2.

Bcl2 belongs to a family of cellular proteins that regulate programmed cell death or apoptosis. The members of this family of proteins perform their function is pairs — either with themselves (e.g. Bcl2-Bcl2) or with other members (e.g. Bcl2-BAX). (Again, I will deliberately avoid going into the jargon or scientific details so that the layperson can understand the discussion.) The relationship of these pairs is a logical one, like switches. If Bcl2 is anti-apoptosis or pro-life (−) and BAX is pro-apoptotic or pro-death (+), then Bcl2-Bcl2 (−/−) twins are anti-apoptotic (i.e. oncogenic). By contrast BAX-BAX (+/+) twins are pro-apoptotic and Bcl2-BAX (−/+) hybrids are balanced, neutral and functionless. With regard to the binding of Ku86v-C and Bcl2 protein, we postulate the following:

- That Ku86v-C could be considered a "member" of the Bcl2 family of proteins.
- That Ku86v-C primarily produces anti-apoptosis (−).

The postulated Ku86v-C-Bcl2 relationship is an anti-apoptotic (−/−) one because of the following. During the CD40 triggering of MM cells, Ku86v-C is found in the cell membrane during the most active phases of cell division. Moreover, Ku86v-C-Bcl2 molecular complexes can actually be isolated from cell membrane extracts of CD40-triggered MM cells and not from non-CD40-triggered MM cells. In fact, preliminary data have suggested that Ku86v-C purified from Ku86v-C-Bcl2 complexes have such a bizarre structure that it is very likely to have gained some novel function, e.g. mimicking the Bcl2 family of proteins. Accordingly, although I do not have absolute proof that Ku86v-C is oncogenic, circumstantial evidence suggests that Ku86v-C could be a putative oncoprotein that promotes anti-apoptosis and cellular longevity. Research is ongoing to prove this and whether the combined effects of both Ku86v-N and Ku86v-C could be even more malicious than either one alone. If indeed so, then development of anti-Ku86v therapies (e.g. mAbs) could be considered for the treatment of MM in the future.

Bone Marrow Microenvironment

Fragility of MM Cells

It might come as a surprise to you to know that cancer cells are actually very fragile cells; especially when they are removed from the bodies that were hosts to them. We are all familiar with how nasty cancers can be, sometimes to point of outright fear. It would seem inconceivable that cancer cells are in fact very delicate living things. The important factor governing a cancer cell's survival is its environment; also call its microenvironment or the tumor bed. Those of us who remember the story, the War of the Worlds, will be able to draw some analogy to this unique requirement of cancer cells. Whilst Martians are portrayed as being indeed strong and sinister, they progressively weaken when removed from their regular environment in Mars. They succumb to agents that are invisible to the naked eye. In a similar way, when MM cells are separated from their "planet," the BM microenvironment, they become almost helpless in their ability to survive and die extremely rapidly. In fact, amongst cancers, this fragility of MM cells outside the body is quite extreme.

Cancer cells that survive for a long time outside the body and in a laboratory are known as cancer cell lines. They are usually grown or cultured in a very special liquid mixture known as a cell culture medium. There are numerous types of cell culture media for various types of cancer cell lines. Certain cancer cell lines can survive in cell culture media that are minimally fortified; but others require more complex and sophisticated media formulations. Although human cancer cell lines can be engineered by genetic manipulations of normal cells in the laboratory, by far, the majority of cancer cell lines are the products of meticulous cell culturing methods of tumor tissue that had been removed from patients with cancer. Interestingly, MM cells are amongst the most difficult types of human cancer cell lines to develop.[29] For the past 50 to 60 years, literally only a handful of MM cell lines were ever successfully established. This was not because no one tried, but that the success rate was well below 1%. In fact, this statistic could qualify MM as the record holder in the Guinness Book of Records for the most difficult cancer for cancer cell line production. The logical conclusion of all this is that the BM microenvironment is an absolute requirement for MM to survive and grow. The BM microenvironment obviously provides all the necessary and critical factors for the cancer to live and behave like a cancer.

Hunting for That Critical Factor

Sometimes, taking a step back helps us see things differently. Instead of hunting in the microscopic world of cells and the insides of cells (the DNA, proteins and organelles), having a bird's eye view of things provides us with more information. The logic is as follows:

- Obviously, MM cells need the comforts of their home, the BM microenvironment to survive and grow.
- The BM microenvironment is found inside bones.
- There must be something about the BM and/or bones that drives the cancerous processes in MM.

Fortunately, a wood etching of a patient with MM that was made about 150 years ago was found. The patient, a middle-aged woman, died from untreated MM. The wood etching depicted the patient in the advanced stages of her disease as suffering from severe bone disease with multiple indiscriminately located fractures. The places where the fractures were found suggested that trauma was not the cause; rather these fractures could have arisen from the most trivial of events. Fractures of this nature are called pathological fractures and suggest a breach of the normal architecture of bones. Other wood etchings of the same patient indeed demonstrated the extensive disease inside the bones had totally damaged its internal architecture. The normal bony cylinder and lacy marrow interior appeared to be completely disrupted and filled with both

104   *Towards Individualized Therapy for Multiple Myeloma*

cancerous tissue as well as other substances. It is not difficult to conclude that the cancerous processes in MM affected not only the BM but also bone itself. This concurs with the symptom complex of patients with MM, i.e. bone pain (without the presence of any fracture) is the commonest symptom experienced by patients with MM. Hence, the critical factor appeared to involve bone itself, and not just the BM.

Although we generally view the skeleton as though it is a fixed and lifeless structure in the body, bone is in fact a living organ. Perhaps it is not as flexible as the heart or the muscles; and certainly not as fluid as blood. Nonetheless, it is as much alive as all our organs. There are, in a simplistic form, 3 parts to our bones:

- The mineral part of bone, called the bone matrix, is perhaps the easiest to appreciate.
- There are bone cells (called osteoblasts, OB) inside this bone matrix that lay down bone.
- And there are bone cells (called osteoclasts, OC) also inside the bone matrix that remove bone.

The laying down of bone is also called bone deposition; and the removal of bone is also called bone resorption. The opposing functions of OBs and OCs lead to a process called bone remodeling and it goes on continuously in our bodies. Because a balance is reached between bone deposition and bone resorption, our bones remain in a normal healthy state, i.e. there is a normal bone matrix content. Bone remodeling is especially important when we sustain fractures as it is the way the body heals itself. This is clearly not the case in MM. Instead, there is a tremendous and virtually complete inhibition of bone deposition and activation of bone resorption. In fact bone resorption goes on relentlessly, leading to complete destruction of the normal bone matrix. As you can easily imagine, the bone architecture is destroyed and thinned out, thus eliminating the supportive function of the bone. Pathological fractures ensue and these may not even heal. As mentioned above, OB function is totally inhibited in established cases of MM; whereas OC function is greatly increased to the point of causing disease.[30–32] In other words, the cancerous processes in MM are suppressive to the OBs and shut down their activity; whereas they are permissive to the OCs and stimulate their activity. The end result is severe destructive bone resorptive and OC-driven bone disease in MM.

Of Mice and OCs

Many researchers in the past tried to create MM in mice by injecting foreign substances (e.g. pristane) that would induce a plasma cell reaction. Interestingly, whilst they were able to induce a plasma cell tumor (also called a plasmacytoma) in these mice, they were by and large unable to create a disease that resembled human MM, which was characterized by intense bony destruction. Similarly, injection of human MM cell lines into experimental mice also often only resulted in the development of single plasmacytomas and not the bony disease of human MM. It appeared that there was a requirement for human bone (especially the OCs) and the human BM microenvironment for the development of MM.

Between 1995 and 1997, I was fortunate to be involved in an experiment that provided us with a critical piece of information in the jigsaw puzzle of MM. Full credit must first go to Professor Kenneth Anderson of the Dana-Farber Cancer Institute, Harvard Medical School in Boston, who was my supervisor at that time. Experimental mice with severe immune deficiency were used in this experiment. These mice were also called severe combined immunodeficiency (SCID) mice and had complete deficiencies of both of the major pathways of specific immunity. These were the specific immunities that were mediated by cells (i.e. cell-mediated immunity) and that were mediated by the liquid parts of the body fluids, e.g. antibodies (i.e. humoral-mediated immunity). The human equivalent of this is David, the "bubble-boy," who lived in an enclosed environment away from germs that would kill him so easily. An important aspect of SCID mice is that immunity was so poor in these mice that if foreign cancer cells were to be injected into these mice, tumors would form. Moreover, even if non-cancerous tissue were implanted into these SCID mice, these tissues would not be rejected and would continue to survive inside the mice.

So, SCID mice were used in an experiment that attempted to recreate human MM disease in a living mouse.[33] Briefly, pieces of normal human bone containing human BM were first implanted into both right and left flanks of SCID mice, just beneath the skin. The end results were SCID mice carrying normal human bones and BM; so-called SCID-hu mice. After the SCID-hu mice recovered from surgery, human MM cells were injected into the region of one of the bone grafts and observed. Amazingly MM tumors formed not only in the region of the injection but also in the bone graft on the other side that was not injected. In other words, the MM disease was now not a single plasmacytoma but a cancer that was occurring in multiple sites. In fact, even the bones of the skeleton of the SCID-hu mice developed tumors. Thus the disease that was created in mice was human MM. This was the first mouse model of human MM that was ever developed.

Around about the same period of time (1996 to 1997), I was reviewing published literature about the BM microenvironment and MM, and there were a number of reports that stated that direct cell-to-cell contact or crosstalk was important in propagating the survival and growth of MM cells. These cell-to-cell communications were thought to be related to multiple cell adhesion molecules that were found on the surface cell membranes of cells, as well as non-cellular substances in the BM microenvironment called the ECM. It was not entirely clear which cell was involved and we simply called the whole group the BM stromal cells (BMSC) to define that they were not of blood origin. The BMSCs included of course the OBs and OCs. An interesting function of BMSCs was their capacity to secrete substances that regulated cell growth. These substances were called growth factors (or cytokines), for want of a better name. Amongst these growth factors that were produced in the BM microenvironment, is a substance called IL-6. As mentioned earlier in the book, IL-6 is the most potent growth factor that mediated survival and proliferation of MM cells. Moreover, the greatest producers of IL-6 in the BM microenvironment were none other than the OCs. Could we have found the villain? Could a normal cell (i.e. OCs are not cancer cells) do so much damage in MM?

Interaction of MM Cells and Osteoclasts

Prior studies have found that direct cell-to-cell interaction of MM cells with OCs is required for the development of MM (Fig. 6.10).[34] The binding of MM cells to the OCs results directly in the following:

- Activation and proliferation of OCs.[35,36]
- Increased bone resorption and development of MM bone disease.
- Production of cytokines, including IL-6, by the OCs.

As mentioned above, IL-6 is the chief growth factor of MM cells. Hence, MM-OC binding eventually (indirectly) leads to increased MM cell survival and proliferation, further MM-OC interactions, and so on and so forth. Because MM-OC cell-to-cell binding is

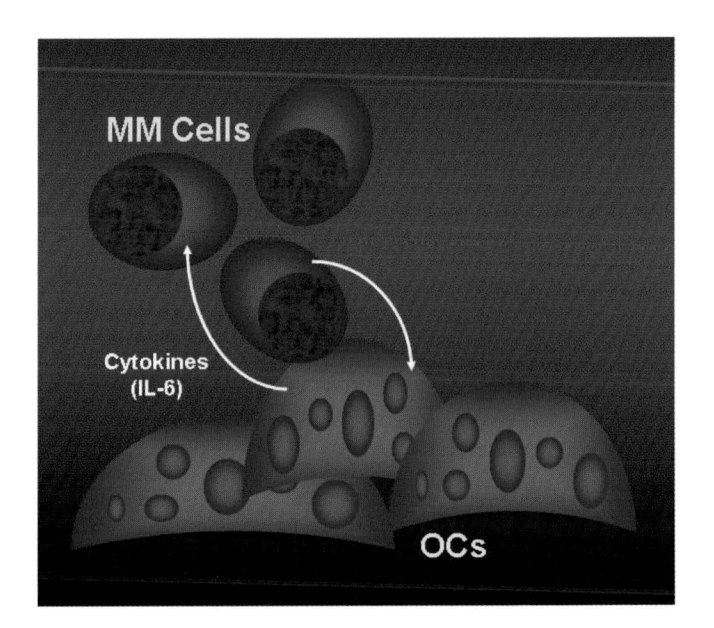

Fig. 6.10. MM-OC interaction.

Towards Individualized Therapy for Multiple Myeloma

required for MM to develop, drugs that are toxic to OCs may have a benefit in the treatment of MM. You will notice that the treatment in this case is not against the MM cell but against a normal non-cancerous cell that participates very actively in the development of MM. In other words, treatment is directed against the collaborating BM microenvironment. Although there are several agents that can be used to eliminate OCs in the bone, none are as potent as a bisphosphonate (or more specifically, an aminobisphosphonate) drug called zoledronic acid (Zometa). This is an interesting drug because it has a chemical structure that resembles the chemical structure of the bone matrix. Because of this similarity, zoledronic acid has a high propensity to be deposited onto bone. The affinity for bone is so high that within one hour of injection, nearly the entire dose is in the bone, and a single injection of the drug can remain in the bone for a year. In the bone, OCs take up zoledronic acid and undergo apoptosis.

Prior studies using the SCID-hu mouse model of MM which I described earlier have confirmed the notion that removal of OCs from the BM microenvironment eliminates MM (i.e. induces an anti-MM effect).[37] There are two types of experiments that are performed, a prevention experiment and a treatment experiment (Table 6.4). Importantly, in both experiments, only zoledronic acid

Table 6.4. Zoledronic Acid's Effects in the SCID-hu Mouse Model of MM

	Prevention Experiment	**Treatment Experiment**
Purpose	Whether removal of OCs will prevent MM from developing	Whether progressive removal of OCs will inhibit MM survival and growth; and eradicate MM
Preparation	SCID-hu mice only	SCID-hu mice with MM tumors
Zoledronic Acid	Single dose	Weekly doses
Observation	Inject MM cells then observe if MM develops	Observe if MM tumors shrink
Result	MM does not develop	MM tumors grew very much slower

was used, so the anti-MM effects are due to zoledronic acid and no other agent.

In the prevention experiment, the question is whether removal of OCs will prevent the development of MM. The SCID-hu mice in this part of the experiment have not been injected with any MM cells. Accordingly, there are no human cancer cells in the body of the mouse. In other words, the effect of zoledronic acid is on the OCs in the human bone chip. After the injection of a single dose of zoledronic acid, human OCs in the bone chip are eliminated and once this has been achieved, live human MM cells are injected into the human bone chip. Indeed, the experiment is successful and MM does not develop in mice pre-treated with zoledronic acid. By contrast, SCID-hu mice that were injected with saline developed MM as saline does not remove OCs. These data confirm the absolute importance of the MM-OC interaction in the development of human MM in a live animal. In fact this experiment is so compelling because it is as close as it can get to a "human" experiment; a point worth noting.

In the treatment experiment, the question is different. It is now whether a SCID-hu mouse that already has MM can be treated and eradicated of MM using a drug that seemingly does not affect the tumor cells but the non-cancerous OCs of the BM microenvironment. In other words, we are not only avoiding the cancer cell as a target, we are eliminating a normal cell. Indeed the results of the treatment experiment demonstrate that MM cell growth is significantly inhibited by zoledronic acid as compared to control mice that were injected with saline. It is worthwhile noting that the inhibition of MM cell growth was not accompanied by total elimination of MM. This is important because the data suggests that although MM-OC interaction may be important in the initial development of MM, OCs might not play such a great role in the later stages of MM when the disease is more established. However, OCs do indeed contribute to the growth of established MM tumors and drugs like zoledronic acid certainly have an important role to play in the total treatment of MM.

110   *Towards Individualized Therapy for Multiple Myeloma*

These experiments in SCID-hu mice provide us with a very firm basis for using anti-OC drugs like zoledronic acid to target the BM microenvironment and treat MM. Not only is the recommendation very logical, it should actually be preferred since MM is clearly a disease that affects the bones. The next logical step is of course to use zoledronic acid in treating humans. Unfortunately, zoledronic acid adversely affects kidney function and about a third of patients with MM have some degree of poor kidney function because of the complications of the disease. As a result, doses of zoledronic acid have to be adjusted to (i) prevent kidney disease and (ii) avoid worsening of kidney function in patients who already have pre-existing kidney problems. It is not difficult to imagine that it is possible to compromise on anti-OC effects when these dose adjustments are made.

Using Zoledronic Acid to Target the BM Microenvironment in Humans

The saying, "Humans are not mice, and mice are not humans" again holds true. In the experiments in SCID-hu mice, the dose of zoledronic acid that was safely used was equivalent (by body weight) to that of a 70-kg man given 8.0 mg of zoledronic acid.

However, in clinical trials in humans, perhaps for reasons of safety, both 4.0 mg and 8.0 mg doses of zoledronic acid were used (Table 6.5). Unfortunately, when 8.0 mg of zoledronic acid was given as a single dose, it was found to cause kidney problems (also called nephrotoxicity) in a small but statistically significant group of

Table 6.5. Use of Zoledronic Acid in Human Clinical Trials — Dose Considerations

Zoledronic Acid	MM	Solid Tumors
4.0 mg	Safe	Safe
8.0 mg	Nephrotoxic in some study arm stopped	Nephrotoxic in some study arm stopped

patients. Zoledronic acid nephrotoxicity was not confined to patients with MM; it was also seen in patients with breast cancer, prostate cancer and other cancers. Hence, it was decided that the safest single dose of zoledronic acid was 4.0 mg and that 8.0 mg of zoledronic acid given as one dose was best avoided. Accordingly, data could only be analyzed for toxicity and not outcome.[38]

This reduction of the dose of zoledronic acid from 8.0 mg to 4.0 mg, i.e. to half of that used in animal studies, produced different results in MM patients and in patients with the other solid tumors (Table 6.6). Whereas a significant benefit is observed in the solid tumors, this phenomenon was clearly missing in MM patients. Indeed, it was rather ironic to see that the cancer in which OCs play the greatest role is now seemingly not responsive to the most potent anti-OC drug. One would have expected the responsiveness of MM to zoledronic acid to be exquisite; but this was clearly not to be. The only possible explanation is that the biology of bone lesions in MM and the other solid tumors must be different. From a broad perspective, MM bone disease is behaving more as a primary event whereas bone lesions in solid tumors are by nature secondary metastatic deposits. If one considers the nature of cancer bone disease from this angle, it becomes clearer that a 4.0 mg dose of zoledronic acid could be inadequate to handle a somewhat "primary" bone disease, as opposed to lesion in the bone that results from the spreading of the cancer from another site. How then can the dose of zoledronic acid be increased to achieve an anti-MM effect?

Table 6.6. Use of Zoledronic Acid in Human Clinical Trials — Efficacy

	MM	Solid Tumors
Risk Benefit for Prevention of Skeletal Related Events	Improved but not statistically significant	Significant improvement
Tumor Burden	Reduction but not statistically significant	Significant reduction
Bone Disease	Primary problem	Secondary event
Zoledronic Acid 4.0 mg	Insufficient	Adequate

112 *Towards Individualized Therapy for Multiple Myeloma*

Equivalent Dose of Zoledronic Acid According to the Size of the Individual

One of my most interesting observations on the dose of zoledronic acid was in the very first patient that I had prescribed zoledronic acid to. This was a man who had failed chemotherapy and was undergoing salvage therapy for relapsed/refractory MM using high-dose dexamethasone. He was suffering from a considerable amount of pain from both MM bone disease as well as from the use of dexamethasone (i.e. glucocorticoid-induced osteoporosis). He had tried all sorts of medicines, including pamidronate (Aredia), a less potent close cousin of zoledronic acid. I offered this patient a trial sample of zoledronic acid (provided by Novartis Oncology), which was at that time a newly-launched drug. Approximately 15 minutes after completion of his zoledronic acid injection, this man returns to my clinic beaming from ear to ear. He told me that he could feel the pain go away even during the injection. This was the first time in months that he had become relatively pain-free. Needless to say, he continued to improve after that and even achieved remission. At the time of writing, this patient had survived beyond six years. The most interesting thing about him was his small stature. He was barely five-feet (1.47 m) tall and weighed only about 40 kg; giving him a body surface area (BSA) of 1.28 m². If the dose of zoledronic acid is 4.0 mg for a person of BSA of 1.82 m² (1.7 m tall and weight 70 kg), the equivalent dose of zoledronic acid in this patient is in fact 5.7 mg, i.e. 5.7 EQmg.

For the less scientific amongst us, this is what it means. If an average-sized individual receives 4.0 mg of zoledronic acid, then a smaller-sized individual receiving 4.0 mg of zoledronic acid is actually receiving more zoledronic acid for his weight when compared to the person of average size. This dose of zoledronic acid is not the actual dose, but a mathematical equivalent based on the standard 4.0 mg dose, and is designated by the unit, EQmg (Table 6.7). Similarly, a larger person will have a smaller dose equivalent than the average person. The effect of this is that patients in reality have their own individual equivalent doses of zoledronic acid – a 4.0 mg

Multiple Myeloma   113

Table 6.7.   Dose Equivalence (EQmg) of Zoledronic Acid

	Weight (kg)	Height (m)	BSA (m^2)	Zoledronic Acid (EQmg)
Small Person	50	1.50	1.44	5.0
Average Person	70	1.70	1.82	4.0
Large Person	90	1.90	2.18	3.3

infusion might be optimal for a smaller person (5.0 EQmg) and grossly insufficient in a larger individual (3.3 EQmg).

Achieving >4.0 EQmg of Zoledronic Acid

Although the 4.0 mg monthly dose of zoledronic acid appears to be inadequate for inducing an anti-MM effect and 8.0 EQmg appears to be sufficient in SCID-hu mice, the actual monthly dose of zoledronic acid for human is still anyone's guess. The maximum dose for a single injection of zoledronic acid is currently 4.0 mg. In the presence of minimal poor kidney function, doses below 4.0 mg (as low as 3.0 mg) are recommended. The peak dose-rate of administration, rather than the total monthly dose of zoledronic acid, appears to be the cause of nephrotoxicity. Hence, achieving doses higher than 4.0 mg is potentially simple with shorter intervals between doses.

According to its product label, zoledronic acid can be prescribed as a single 4.0 mg dose as frequently as 3-weekly, provided that kidney function is normal. Over a period of two months or approximately 63 days, 12.0 mg of zoledronic acid can be given (Table 6.8). This works out to be approximately 6.0 EQmg a month and is the maximum recommended dosing rate of zoledronic acid.

When we now apply the effect of body size to the dosing rate of zoledronic acid, we find that even for larger persons, 3-weekly dosing increases the equivalent dose to greater than 4.0 EQmg/month (Table 6.9). And for smaller persons, the equivalent dose is nearly 8.0 EQmg/month. Hence, higher frequency or 3-weekly dosing of zoledronic acid is highly desirable as it is more likely to produce an anti-MM effect.

114　*Towards Individualized Therapy for Multiple Myeloma*

Table 6.8. Dose Equivalence (EQmg) of 3-Weekly and Monthly Zoledronic Acid

Zoledronic Acid	3-Weekly	Monthly
Injection Dose (mg)	4.0	4.0
Base Rate	4.0 mg/21 days	4.0 mg/30 days
Total Dose for ~60 days (mg)	~4.0 × 3 = ~12.0	4.0 × 2 = 8.0
Monthly Dose Rate (EQmg)	~6.0	4.0

Table 6.9. Effect of Body Size on Dosing Rate of Zoledronic Acid

	BSA (m²)	3-Weekly (EQmg/month)	Monthly (EQmg/month)
Small Person	1.44	~7.5	5.0
Average Person	1.82	~6.0	4.0
Large Person	2.18	~5.0	3.3

Ultra-High Dose Rate Zoledronic Acid

As discussed above, human clinical trials using zoledronic acid for the treatment of MM have demonstrated potent activity in bone healing and prevention of skeletal related events (SRE).[39] Despite compelling preclinical data,[40,41] an anti-MM effect has never been demonstrated in humans due to differences in the doses of zoledronic acid that were administered to either animals or humans.[42] Serendipitously, we had the opportunity of studying three patients with MM who received two to three doses of zoledronic acid within a period of 28 days, i.e. an ultra-high dose rate of zoledronic acid. Interestingly, these rapid doses of zoledronic acid were not given for inducing an anti-MM effect, but for control of intractable hypercalcemia and refractory bone pain that were only controlled by zoledronic acid. What caught our eye after these infusions were the brisk clinical anti-MM responses. In fact, one patient even achieved a sustained immunofixation (IF)-negative complete remission (CR) of over six years at the time of the writing of this book. I believe that these favorable clinical observations were attributable, at least

Table 6.10. Ultra-high Dose Rate of Zoledronic Acid

	BSA (m^2)	EQmg	Maximum Monthly Doses	Maximum Dosing Rate (EQmg^{max}/28d)	Clinical Outcome
Patient 1	1.27	5.7	2	11.4	Near complete remission
Patient 2	1.28	5.7	2	11.4	Complete remission
Patient 3	1.82	4.0	3	12.0	Substantial decrease in peripheral blood plasma cells

in part, to the use of ultra-high dose rate of zoledronic acid because a number of other patients have also achieved good results with a similar dosing frequency.

The effects of the three patients who were treated with ultra-high (i.e. more frequent than 3-weekly) dosing of zoledronic acid are summarized in Table 6.10 above. When the equivalent dose (EQmg) of zoledronic acid was adjusted to the body surface area, the maximum EQmg rate of Zol administered was between 11.4 EQmg^{max} to 12.0 EQmg^{max} per 28 days. Mild, reversible hypocalcemia was observed in two patients. Renal function was significantly ($p < 0.001$) improved in all three patients. These data suggest that the anti-tumor effect of zoledronic acid in MM could be dose-rate-dependent. Moreover, delivery of high dose-rate zoledronic acid may be achieved by judiciously increasing the monthly dosing frequency of zoledronic acid.

Patient 1

The first patient is a 61-year-old Chinese woman (body surface area, BSA 1.27 m^2; 5.7 EQmg zoledronic acid) with a newly diagnosed, ISS stage II, non-secretory MM, who also had diabetes mellitus with mild PNY (Fig. 6.11). Because of poor performance status and PNY, we elected not to give chemotherapy, glucocorticoids or thalidomide, but instead only to treat conservatively with zoledronic acid (i.e. monotherapy). Since body movement provoked episodes of severe pain, a second dose of zoledronic acid was infused three

116 *Towards Individualized Therapy for Multiple Myeloma*

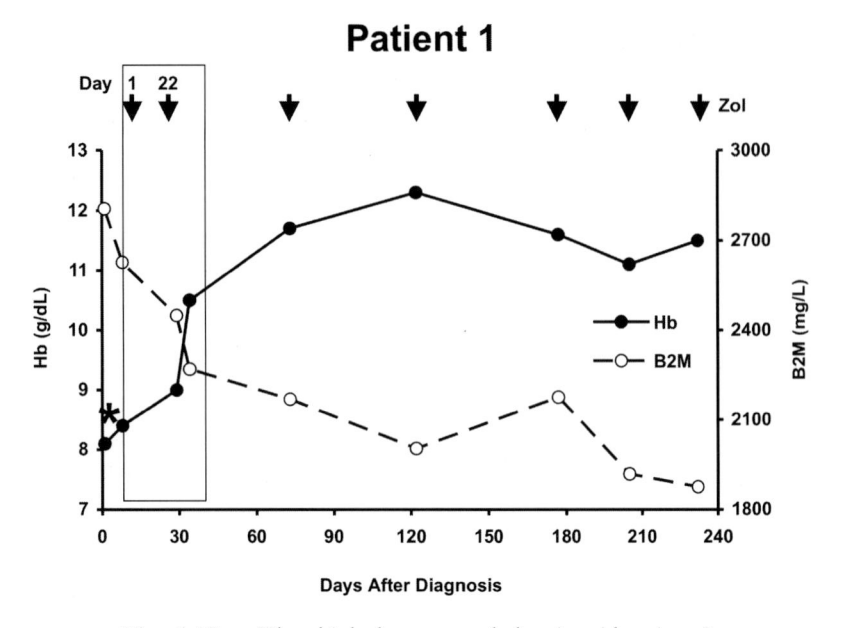

Fig. 6.11.   Ultra-high dose rate zoledronic acid patient 1.

weeks (day 22) after the first. Unfortunately, we had a slight difficulty analyzing this patient because she had a non-secretory MM.
In a small percentage of MM patients, the malignant plasma cells do
not produce the abnormal M-protein. This means that we cannot
specifically track the disease with absolute accuracy. If we were able
to perform regular repeated BM examinations, that could be a way
of tracking disease response. However, this is understandably very
challenging to both patient and doctor. Instead, we use surrogate
markers, including the hemoglobin (Hb) and B2M. The B2M is a
well-known marker of the tumor burden in MM[43,44]; and the Hb is
used to support the changes observed in the B2M. I would like to
point out that a single (blood) transfusion of packed red cells
(Fig. 6.11 asterisk) raised the Hb from 8.1 g/dL to 8.4 g/dL, and
did not affect our analysis. As can be seen in Fig. 6.11, zoledronic
acid monotherapy was associated with normalization of B2M and
improved Hb levels. Since the greatest improvements in B2M and
Hb occurred during the period when the maximum dose rate of
zoledronic acid (11.4 EQmg^{max}/28 days) was administered (Fig. 6.11
box), these data suggest that the anti-MM effect of zoledronic acid

Multiple Myeloma 117

could be dose rate-dependent. Moreover, we also noted the complete recovery of initially depressed levels of normal IgM which occurred maximally during the 28-day window of time (data not shown). Importantly, kidney function was not significantly compromised. Furthermore, no serious side effects (e.g. low calcium levels (hypocalcemia) or a serious abnormality called osteonecrosis of the jaw(s) (ONJ)[45-47] that causes the jaw bones to break down and become dead) were seen.

Patient 2

The next patient is a 76-year-old Chinese woman (BSA 1.28 m^2; 5.7 EQmg zoledronic acid) with ISS stage III IgGκ POEMS syndrome (Fig. 6.12). The POEMS syndrome consists of:

- Polyneuropathy — abnormalities of the nerves to the limbs

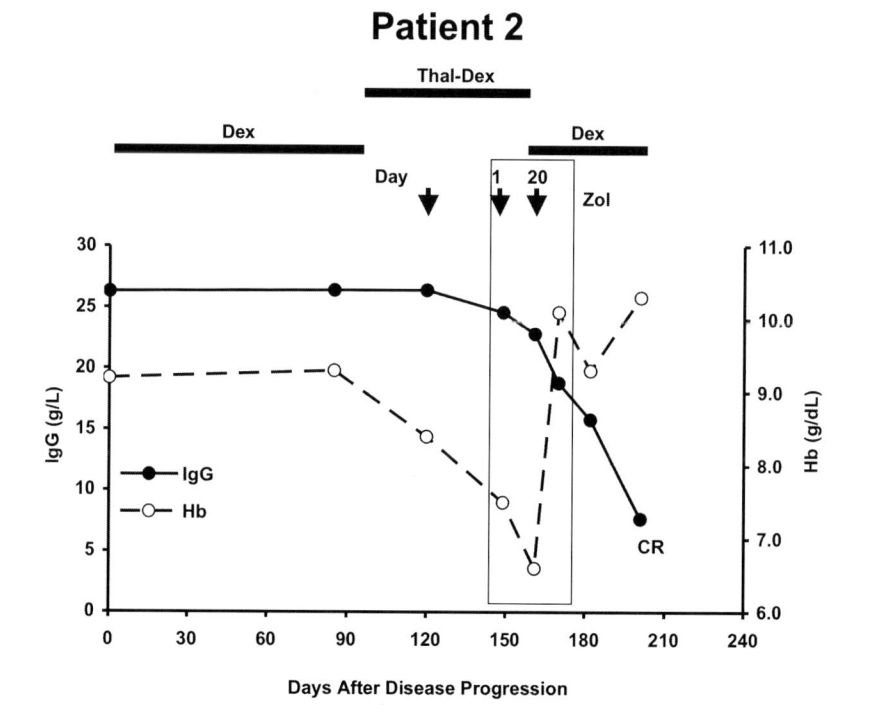

Fig. 6.12. Ultra-high dose rate zoledronic acid patient 2.

- Organomegaly — enlargement of some of the organs of the body (e.g. lymph nodes)
- Endocrinopathy — disturbances in the hormones of the body (e.g. thyroid problems)
- M-Protein — MM
- Skin Changes — usually increased skin thickening or hairiness

Over the past 11 years, she had received numerous cycles of combination chemotherapy and/or pulsed glucocorticoids. She was in a stable disease (plateau) phase for three years when her disease started to progress. Because she was having very low blood counts (pancytopenia) and was considered unsuitable for further chemotherapy, we elected to treat her with dexamethasone (Dex) and later on thalidomide (Thal) (50 mg orally twice a week to 50 mg every night at bedtime) as well. An additional dose of zoledronic acid was infused within three weeks of the first dose (day 20) because she had severe bone pain. As can be seen in Fig. 6.12 Day 120, a modest fall in the IgG M-protein level was observed when zoledronic acid was first administered. Thereafter, progressive reduction in IgG M-protein levels accompanied by rapid recovery of the Hb followed the use of additional doses of zoledronic acid (Fig. 6.12, box). Remarkably, this previously dexamethasone-resistant patient continued to show progressive recovery and eventually achieved an IF-negative complete response (CR). Similar to the first patient, the maximum dose rate of zoledronic acid was 11.4 EQmg^{max}/28 days. These data suggest that ultra-high dose rate zoledronic acid could produce a significant anti-MM effect, even to the point of CR. The only side effect experience by this patient was a mild, transient hypocalcemia, which was readily reversed with intravenous calcium gluconate. Importantly, renal function was not compromised but significantly improved. This patient also did not develop ONJ.

Patient 3

The third patient is a 48-year-old Chinese man (BSA 1.82 m²; 4.0 EQmg zoledronic acid) who presented at 11 months with an

Multiple Myeloma 119

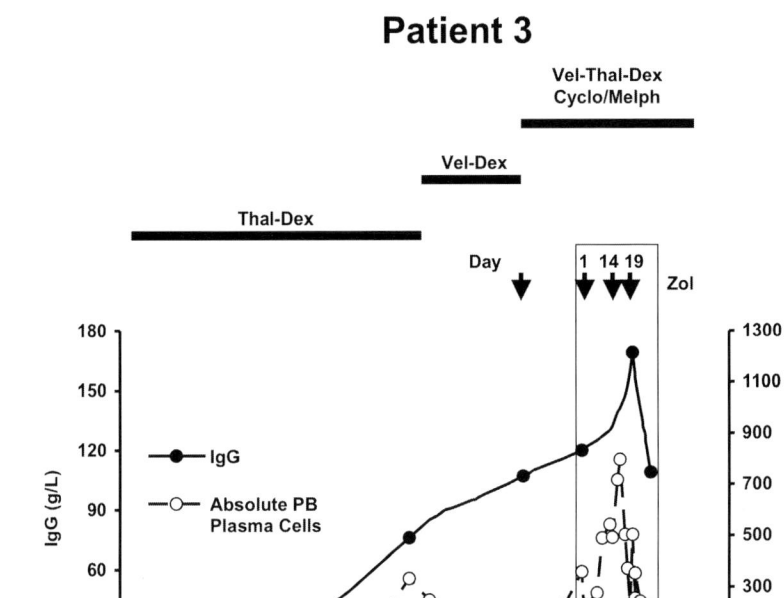

Fig. 6.13. Ultra-high dose rate zoledronic acid patient 3.

ISS stage III IgGκ plasma cell leukemia (PCL) (Fig. 6.13). The genetic profile (karyotype) of his MM cells contained complex chromosomal (cytogenetic) abnormalities, including a much dreaded gene signature called deletion of chromosome 13 (del(13)). He received six cycles of standard chemotherapy, consisting of VAD chemotherapy over eight months and achieved a partial response (PR). Unfortunately, his disease continued to worsen within three months of completing VAD chemotherapy and he was changed to targeted therapies, i.e. monthly cycles of Thal-Dex. The pace of disease progression continued to accelerate and treatment was changed to bortezomib (Velcade)-Dex for 2 cycles.[51] Treatment was intensified using two cycles of Velcade-Thal-Dex with cyclophosphamide (100 mg orally on days 1, 4, 8 and 11) and zoledronic acid (4.0 mg IV on day 1); and then one cycle of Velcade-Thal-Dex with melphalan (8 mg orally on days 1, 4, 8 and 11). Two additional doses of zoledronic acid were administered (on days 14 and 19 of the second cycle of Velcade-Thal-Dex-Cyclophosphamide) because of severe bone pain. Following the first two doses of zoledronic acid, two dips in the absolute peripheral blood plasma cell count were noted (Fig. 6.13, asterixes). When two further doses of zoledronic acid were infused in quick succession, on days 14 and 19 of that cycle (Fig. 6.13, box), a rapid fall in the IgG M-protein and absolute peripheral blood plasma cells was observed. The maximal dose rate of zoledronic acid that was achieved was 12.0 EQmg^{max}/ 28 days. These data again suggest that ultra-high dose rate of zoledronic acid could produce an anti-MM effect. There was a mild but slightly prolonged (10 days) hypocalcemia which required intravenous and oral calcium supplements. We attributed this to the combined effects of zoledronic acid on OC inhibition and Velcade on OB activation — which induce a so-called "hungry bone" syndrome. Importantly, kidney function was preserved. This patient also did not develop ONJ.

Conclusions on Ultra-high Dose Rate Zoledronic Acid

These case studies illustrate the following:

- Firstly, that zoledronic acid monotherapy is effective in managing early stage MM; and provides evidence of a clinical anti-MM effect.
- Secondly, that zoledronic acid may be at least additive to or even synergistic with other drugs in mediating tumor rejection.
- Thirdly, that in selected patients, the combined effects of zoledronic acid possibly with another agent could even induce CR.
- Fourthly, that a higher dosing rate of zoledronic acid is required to achieve these effects. Accordingly, it is tempting to speculate that delivering zoledronic acid at a sufficiently high rate (e.g. 4.0 mg twice or thrice a month) could inhibit MM-OC interactions in the BM microenvironment and induce apoptosis of tumor cells.

One is of course concerned about preventing kidney damage and inducing ONJ when zoledronic acid is used at a high dose-rate. Contrary to expectations, there was in fact a statistically significant ($p < 0.001$; Chi-squared test) improvement in kidney function for the whole group. In addition, since prior studies have suggested that it is the longer-term use of bisphosphonates that predisposes to ONJ, the lack of ONJ developing in our patients argues in favor of safety for the administration of ultra-high dose rate zoledronic acid, albeit for a limited period of time. In conclusion, the anti-MM effect of zoledronic acid in MM could possibly be dose rate-dependent. Achieving levels of zoledronic acid that are associated with anti-MM effect is easily and safely done by judiciously increasing the dosing frequency of standard 4.0 mg infusions of zoledronic acid to two to three doses a month over a short period of time. This is especially prudent in situations where potential benefits could far outweigh theoretically perceived risks.

Blood Supply

Without a doubt, in our experience, the key to successful control on MM is in the blood supply. In the blood that supplies the tumor bed or BM microenvironment are cells that will eventually develop into OCs. These pOCs constitute a renewable pool of potentially lethal cells because they eventually feed fresh OCs to the cancerous processes that promote the development of MM. Prior studies using parabiosis[i] experiments have identified these pOCs as PB monocytes. Interestingly, MM-OC contact drives this very process, adding further to the maliciousness of this poorly-recognized circuit.

---

[i] Parabiosis is an experiment involving two living animals. These animals are usually littermates (siblings) that have the ability to share their blood supplies without adverse effects. If one surgically connects their blood supplies (arteries and veins), blood from one animal can freely enter the other littermate, and vice versa. This is called parabiosis. If there is a condition that is present in one littermate and not the other, free exchange of blood may reversibly affect the other after parabiosis is performed.

I have termed this cancerous cellular pathway the "Monocyte Loop" and will elaborate further on how to block it.

"I regard the blockade of the "Monocyte Loop" as the single most important goal in individualized therapy for MM — every effort must be made to steer monocytes away from the blood that supplies the BM microenvironment."

Parabiosis and pOCs

There is a condition called osteopetrosis in which patients are born without any OCs. As you can imagine, osteopetrosis will lead to very hard bones because only bone deposition (the function of OBs) and not bone resorption (the function of OCs) is active. Interestingly, there are mice that suffer from osteopetrosis and since the disease is a genetic and of a dominant nature, 50% of mouse littermates have osteopetrosis and 50% are completely normal. This presents us with a unique opportunity to study OCs and pOCs, especially if we perform a parabiosis experiment. In an incredibly elegant experiment more than 35 years ago, Walker performed precisely the above experiment, a parabiosis between osteopetrotic mice and their normal littermates.[52] Following which, he observed the dramatic and complete repletion of OCs, and resolution of osteopetrosis in all the affected mice and concluded that the PB contained the critical elements or precursors for OC development. Whether these were cellular and/or non-cellular was a mystery until much later when several researchers discovered that these circulating pOCs were actually the PB monocytes.[53,54] The implications of these finding on MM are as follows:

- If there are increased numbers of monocyte pOCs, then there are likely to be even greater numbers of OCs as the pOCs differentiate into OCs.
- If monocyte pOC numbers increase for whatever reason, e.g. cancer-induced release of growth factors/cytokines and infections, these pOCs would eventually feed further into the already expanded OC pool.

- If blood supply were increased through the cancerous process called angiogenesis, then there will be an abundant and ever expanding supply of pOCs.

The "Monocyte Loop"

Whatever the mechanism, the same conclusions are drawn. Peripheral blood monocytes pose a threat to the patient with MM because they induce expansion of the OC compartment. Unfortunately, OCs in MM secrete other cytokines (including monocyte growth factors[55]) that eventually generate more monocytes or pOCs. The vicious cycle is established when MM cells bind to newly-formed OCs in what I call the "Monocyte Loop" (Fig. 6.14). As you can easily imagine, this loop poses a real problem in OC and consequently MM cell control.

Prior reports have shown that MM is frequently accompanied by a certain degree of monocytosis.[56–58] This is illustrated in Fig. 6.15, where the absolute monocyte count (AMCO) of 50 patients with

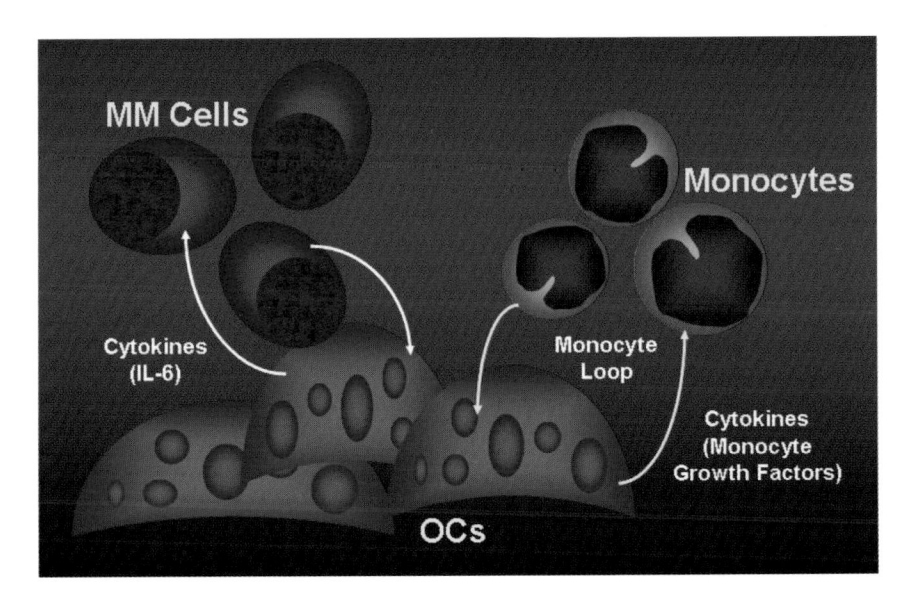

Fig. 6.14.   The "Monocyte Loop".

124   *Towards Individualized Therapy for Multiple Myeloma*

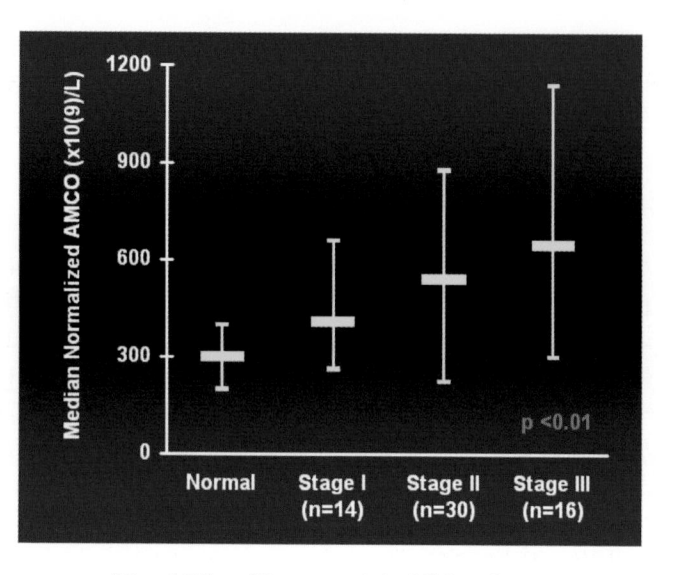

Fig. 6.15.   Monocytosis in MM patients.

MM was correlated with the ISS stage of MM at the time of disease presentation. Indeed there was a statistically significant and almost linear correlation between the ISS stage of MM and the degree of PB monocytosis. Moreover, successful treatment of MM results in lower AMCO levels. The relationship of MM and monocytosis goes even further in that it has been well-recognized that MM occasionally co-exists with the monocytic leukemias.[59-61] The relationship of monocytosis with cancer bone disease is not confined to MM. Peripheral blood monocyte expansion is a dominant feature of late stage cancers (e.g. breast and lung cancer) where the patients have extensive osteolytic bone disease. It has also been reported that osteolytic bone disease can result directly from the activity of pOCs/monocytes without differentiation into OCs.[62]

The inhibitory effects of bisphosphonates and especially the aminobisphosphonates on OCs in MM are well known.[63] Inhibition and inactivation of OCs result in decreased bone resorption and IL-6 production. However, bisphosphonates have also been shown to be at least cytostatic on the MM cells, with the possibility of being cytotoxic as well. Current evidence suggests that the antitumor

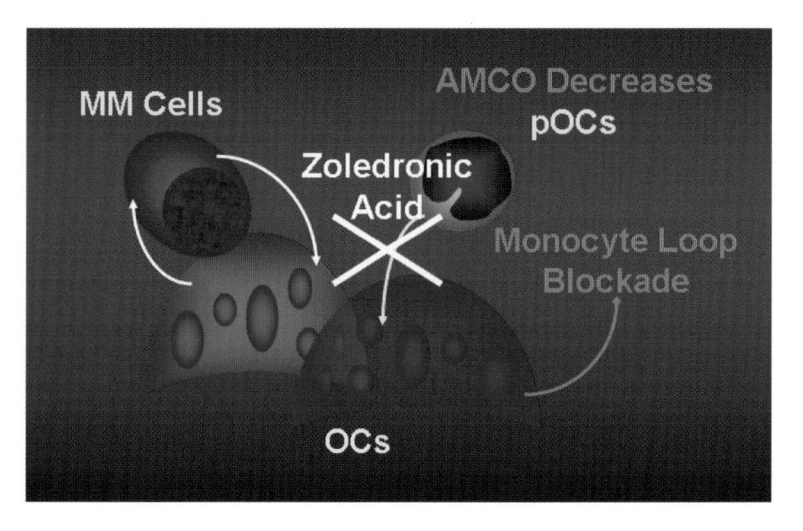

Fig. 6.16. Blockade of the "monocyte loop" by zoledronic acid.

activity of bisphosphonates may be related to the specific chemical structure of the bisphosphonate molecule, rather than to a class effect. In other words, not all bisphosphonates are the same; there are clear differences in potency and one has to be selective when deciding on the bisphosphonate to use. The potency of a bisphosphonate is measured by its ability to inhibit the differentiation of pOCs to OCs (Fig. 6.16). These pre-clinical studies in rats demonstrate that third-generation nitrogen-containing aminobisphosphonates, e.g. pamidronate and zoledronic acid, may be up to 20 to 20 000 times more potent, respectively, than first-generation non-nitrogenous bisphosphonates like clodronate.[64] Accordingly, one would expect that zoledronic acid would be more capable of blocking the "Monocyte Loop" than pamidronate.

In 2005, we analyzed the ability of pamidronate and zoledronic acid in inhibiting AMCO levels in patients with MM (Fig. 6.17). The reported difference in potency, as measured by the ability to block pOC to OC conversion in rats between pamidronate and zoledronic acid, is about three orders of magnitude or 1000-fold. In other words, zoledronic acid was about 1000 times more potent than pamidronate. The clinical study was a very small one, a pilot

126   *Towards Individualized Therapy for Multiple Myeloma*

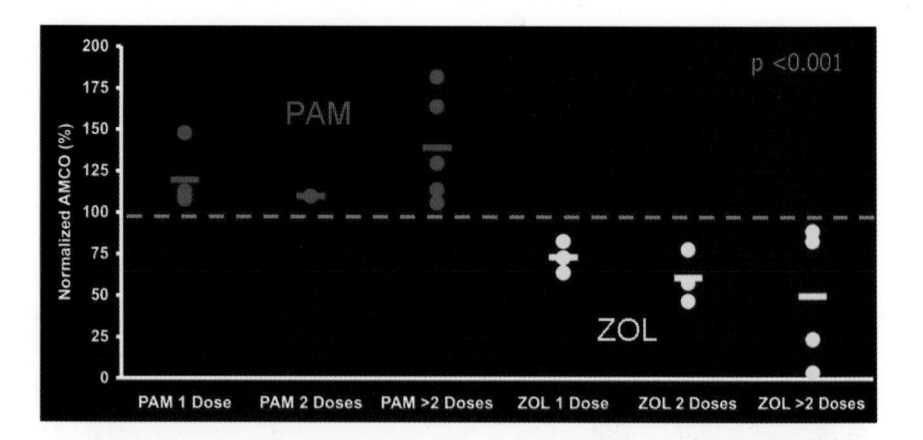

Fig. 6.17.   Dose-dependent "monocyte loop" blockade by zoledronic acid.

study with just 10 patients in each arm. It hoped to demonstrate in clinical terms that the difference in potency of these two amino-bisphosphonates was the reason for their anti-pOC activity. The read-out was the percentage change in the post-treatment AMCO. Apart from the different bisphosphonates that the two groups of patients were given, all other anti-MM drugs were the same, i.e. all patients also received Thal-Dex. As can be seen in Fig. 6.17, there was a significant ($p < 0.001$) reduction of pOCs in patients treated with zoledronic acid; but not in patients treated with pamidronate. Patients treated with pamidronate not only failed to show reduction in the AMCO, it appeared that as they were given more doses of pamidronate, the AMCO levels rose further. In fact, these differences were so striking that we wondered whether pamidronate could have a detrimental effect. By contrast, the decreases in AMCO levels induced by zoledronic acid were well measured and appeared to be dependent on the number of doses administered ($p < 0.001$). These data were fully consistent with our hypothesis of "Monocyte Loop" blockade.

As predicted, the inhibition of pOCs/AMCO was associated with a favorable outcome. Patients who received zoledronic acid (also called DTZOL) fared significantly ($p < 0.001$) better than those who received pamidronate (DTPAM) (Fig. 6.18). This superior clinical

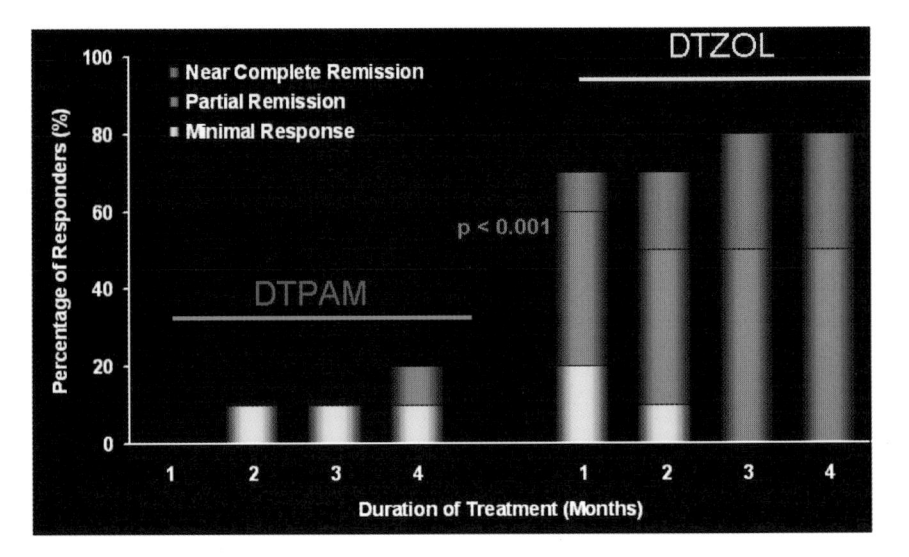

Fig. 6.18. Clinical outcome after "monocyte loop" blockade by zoledronic acid.

outcome could only come about if zoledronic acid exerted a clinical anti-MM effect. We therefore concluded that monocyte-driven OC renewal (the "Monocyte Loop") in MM is inhibited by zoledronic acid (but not by pamidronate) in a dose-dependent fashion; and that this malicious cellular pathway must be effectively blocked in the treatment of MM.

Finally, with all the background information, we tested our hypotheses in a patient (Fig. 6.19). This 78-year-old man had an IgG MM with a greatly elevated paraprotein level of >100 g/L at the time of diagnosis. Because of his age and his very poor clinical state, he was given palliative treatment with melphalan (single-agent oral chemotherapy) plus. The expected RR for this melphalan/ Pred (MP) combination regimen was 45%. In other words, 55% of patients were not expected to respond to it; and this gentleman was one of those non-responders. After about four to five cycles of MP, he was changed to a second-line regimen which consisted of full dose Thal-Dex plus 4-weekly pamidronate (Aredia), or the "DTa" regimen. There was a modest response but the side effects from full doses of Thal and Dex for six cycles made him very sick.

128   *Towards Individualized Therapy for Multiple Myeloma*

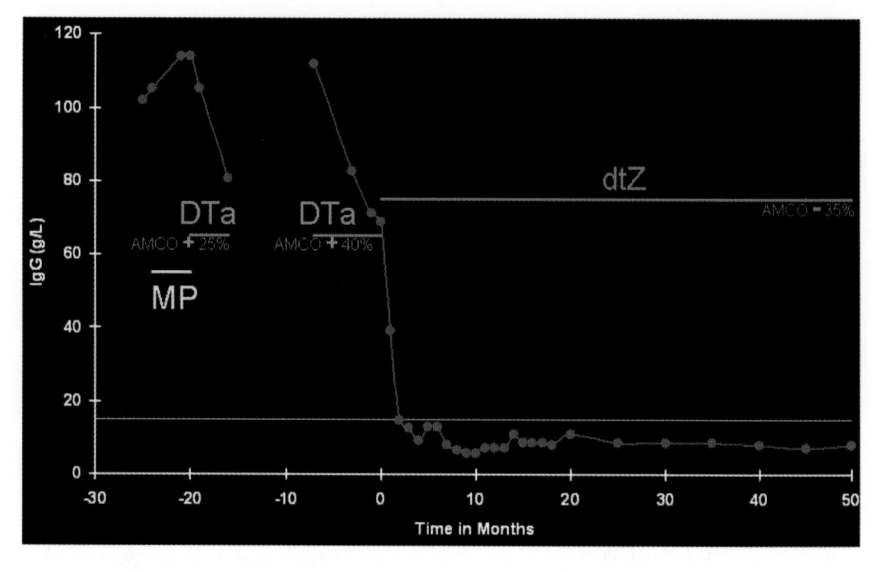

Fig. 6.19.   High-frequency (3-weekly) zoledronic acid — index patient.

He gave up and sought complementary medicine. However, after several months, he returned for treatment because he was not getting any better, and was restarted on "DTa" for another seven cycles. It is worthwhile noting that during both courses of "DTa" the AMCO remained elevated by 25% and 40%, respectively, above the pre-treatment levels.

He was about to throw in the towel a second time when he was transferred to my clinic. I reduced his Thal doses by a whopping 75%, and his Dex doses by 30%; and switched him from 4-weekly pamidronate to 3-weekly zoledronic acid. And because his BSA was smaller than average, his $EQmg^{max}$/month was ~7.0. Within three cycles over nine weeks, he achieved near complete remission (nCR); and he said that he never felt better in his life. From hobbling in pain, he could now walk five km daily for exercise. The most striking change was a decrease in his AMCO by 35% below baseline. This patient's regimen of low doses of Thal-Dex and 3-weekly zoledronic acid became known as the "dtZ" regimen. I followed him up after starting him on "dtZ" for about four years, and he continued to be in good disease control throughout those four years.

There is no doubt in my mind that a high dose rate of zoledronic acid individualized to lower AMCO levels and induce "Monocyte Loop" blockade is fundamental to good clinical outcome. Agents like Thal and Dex facilitate this process by inhibiting neoplastic blood supply (Thal) and further inhibiting monocytes/pOCs (Dex). Other agents like Velcade may assist bone healing by activating OBs, and contribute to therapy.

We should be constantly aware that it is not so much the nutrients in the blood supply that are feeding the myelomagenic process; it is the monocytes/pOCs. Measuring AMCO levels is very simple, it is found in the most routine blood test, the full or complete blood count (FBC or CBC). Above is another patient who had regular FBCs performed on her during follow-up and the changes in her Hb are plotted against the corresponding AMCO level (Fig. 6.20). At about 14 months into treatment, she was given ultra-high dose rate zoledronic acid (~11.5 EQmg^{max}/month) because of persistently elevated AMCO levels. Her AMCO level fell below 200/μL which was associated with good clinical recovery. Thereafter, she was maintained on 3-weekly zoledronic acid and finally achieved CR. As you can see, she had very favorable AMCO levels following

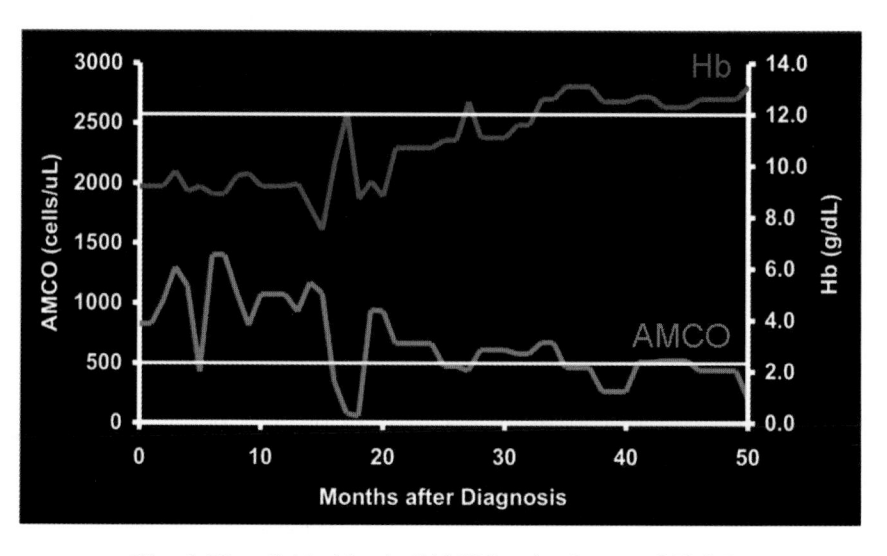

Fig. 6.20. Critical level of AMCO reduction — <200/μL.

130   *Towards Individualized Therapy for Multiple Myeloma*

ultra-high dose rate zoledronic acid. By individualizing therapy for her to achieve the desired AMCO level and "Monocyte Loop" blockade, this patient went on to have a great recovery.

Immune System

Our body's immune system is the defense system against invasion from foreign substances, including bacteria and viruses. Moreover, our immune system is thought to be able to protect us from developing cancer by searching out cancerous cells and eliminating them. The immune system does this efficiently and quietly without us being even aware of its activities. Cancer is thought to develop because our immune system has suffered a system failure and permitted a rather more resilient and tenacious cancer cell to survive and grow. The list is long for the multitude of ways it can do this. Amongst the more current and less appreciated concepts are the so-called Regulatory T cells/lymphocytes (Tregs). Interestingly, the MM cell is a cell of the immune system. Its normal counterpart, the plasma cell, produces antibodies that protect the body from foreign invasion. Hence, MM is a cancer of the immune system itself. In becoming a cancer, MM destroys its own team and induces profound immunity.

The field of immunology is very complex. There is no need for the layperson to delve and get confused by it. I know of many a layman or even a junior doctor who has attempted to understand the immune system. Unfortunately, there is no simple way to do this. Table 6.11 attempts to provide the reader with the most basic structure of the immune system. This alone might already be too complex for some and I really apologize for it. If you are unable to understand it, take heart, you're probably amongst the majority. All that there needs to be said is that all four aspects of the immune system are terribly abnormal in MM. Myeloma is a form of cancer that induces truly deranged immunodeficiency. More specifically, prior studies have demonstrated a profound lack of expression of immune co-stimulatory molecules (especially B7-1) that results in specific T cell anergy and immunoparesis in MM.[65] The recovery of immune function after treatment is an exceptionally good indicator of a favorable clinical outcome.[66]

Multiple Myeloma 131

Table 6.11.   Simple Immunology

	Non-Cellular	Cells
Broad immunity	Substances that have a general protective function, e.g. inducing sticking and punching out holes in cell membranes	Cells that produce substances that digest foreign particles or have a scavenger or housekeeping function
Specific immunity	Antibodies	Killer, Helper & Suppressor Cells

Even though there is widespread suppression of the immune system in most patients with MM, many doctors do not routinely monitor the patient's immune status. This is probably because of the complexity of the immune system and the difficulty in coming to a reasonably good conclusion about the immune status. Adding to this difficulty is the requirement of a fairly high level of sophistication when carrying out such tests; and this level of expertise is not widely and/or commercially available. It is not surprising that assessment of the immunological status, though extremely important, has taken a backseat in the management of patients with MM. However, I am confident that some sensible assessment of immune function can still be made using clinical information as well as some common laboratory investigations (Table 6.12). I would recommend that only in the more serious patient, or when marking treatment milestones, that more sophisticated testing should be performed. Our experiences with the "dtZ" regimen, which does not in any way harm the immune system, has taught us some valuable lessons about immunological assessment in MM. These fairly simple assessments have helped me further individualize therapy for my patients.

Serum Albumin

The ISS for the prognostic risk of MM uses the serum albumin as one of its two parameters (the other being the B2M). Patients with advanced and poor risk MM have low levels of serum albumin.

132 *Towards Individualized Therapy for Multiple Myeloma*

Table 6.12. Some Markers of Immunodeficiency in MM

	Non-Cellular	Cells
Broad immunity	(Albumin) *No really good marker*	Peripheral Blood Absolute Neutrophil Count (ANC)
Specific immunity	Normal Immunoglobulins (IgG, IgA, IgM)	Peripheral Blood Absolute Lymphocyte Count BM Regulatory T Cells (Tregs)

Since albumin is produced in the liver, it is perhaps more of a marker of the health of the liver than of the seriousness of MM. Moreover, in patients with advanced MM and kidney disease, large amounts of albumin can be lost in the urine due to a condition called the nephrotic syndrome. At no point is the serum albumin a direct measure of immune function. So why use it to assess immune function? The reasons are:

- There is really no other readily available marker of broad-based non-cellular immunity
- Low albumin correlates fairly well with poor health; and poorer health by and large implies poorer immunity
- Albumin is a major prognostic factor in MM
- Use it for all its worth, with a good lump of salt

Absolute Neutrophil Count

This parameter is much, much better than the serum albumin. The ANC is a traditional measure of broad-based cellular immunity. Different physicians use different algorithms to manage low ANCs. A simple layman's algorithm could be as follows:

- Below 1500/μL — warning
- Below 1000/μL — isolation required
- Below 500/μL — intervention with growth factors (e.g. granulocyte colony-stimulating factor, G-CSF)

It is not the purpose of this book to discuss low ANCs or the condition termed neutropenia. However, there are two special scenarios concerning the ANC in MM that the patient and/or doctor may need to be aware of:

- **Demargination.** Severe BM suppression by MM can lead to neutropenia. If glucocorticoids (e.g. Dex) are used to treat MM, the ANC can rise sharply because of a phenomenon called demargination. In this condition, glucocorticoids release (demarginate) neutrophils that are bound to the walls of the blood vessels, especially those in the lungs. There is no net increase in neutrophils and the apparent recovery of ANCs is spurious.
- **"Myeloma-Plus" Syndrome.** Some patients with MM have additional hematological problems; what I call a "Myeloma-Plus" syndrome. In other words, MM may not exist alone. Certain genetic signatures are shared between different blood disorders and can hypothetically induce two disorders in close succession. Moreover, the causative events (e.g. exposure to toxic chemicals) may provoke more than one disorder. Logically, MM should not directly affect the ANC. However, when the ANC is affected (usually persistently decreased for no apparent reason), a "Myeloma-Plus" syndrome, such as a Myelodysplastic Syndrome (MDS), should be suspected and investigated for.

Normal IgG, IgA, IgM

This collectively is an interesting and important parameter in assessing the immune status in MM. The usual scenario is as follows:

- At the time of diagnosis, there is a decrease in the levels of the normal Igs
- The logical expectation for treatment of MM is for normal Ig levels to increase back to normal; and for M proteins to decrease to zero
- Since both normal Igs and M proteins (which are cancer Igs) are produced by plasma cells, one benign and one malignant,

treatment of MM will frequently prevent the recovery of normal Igs

- What is frequently observed is the progressive decrease in the M protein level during treatment (which is good), but the failure of the normal Igs to increase.

In reality, this is an expected observation; since normal plasma cells are logically inhibited by anti-MM therapy. What must be realized is that at the late stages of treatment when only low levels of M-protein or tumor burden (e.g. low B2M states) are left, the pursuit of aggressive lines of therapy to eradicate residual disease might actually prove to be counter-productive to immunological recovery. Accordingly, lightening up treatment to permit recovery of normal Igs could prove to be more beneficial for the patient's immune system. There is no doubt that treatment at this stage must be individualized. One does not want to continue suppressive therapy in the face of low tumor burden. The key to decision making is the B2M. If the B2M is low, it is time to wean off treatment (see below).

Absolute Lymphocyte Count

Similar to the ANC, the absolute lymphocyte count is another straightforward parameter that is readily available from the FBC. The absolute lymphocyte count is related to immunity that is specific and of a cellular nature. This kind of immunity is considered highly advanced in the animal kingdom, and humans are certainly very fortunate to have such an excellent system. When individualizing therapy to permit optimal immunological recovery, the absolute lymphocyte count should be kept above 1000/μL. Just like normal plasma cells (which originate from B lymphocytes), normal lymphocytes are also affected by drugs that are used to treat MM cells. Lymphocyte suppression is an expected phenomenon but it is best to "keep the head above the water" and not permit it to fall too low for too long. Permitting the absolute lymphocyte count to dip below 200/μL for a continuous period of two months is nearly always fatal in our experience. The rough rule of thumb to keep above 1000/μL cannot be over-emphasized. If lower levels are unavoidable, prophylactic use of antiviral drugs, e.g. acyclovir (Zovirax), is highly-recommended. When dealing with low lymphocyte counts (lymphopenia), treatment must be individualized.

Bone Marrow Regulatory T Cells

This is a fairly new parameter that surfaced over the past five years. Bone marrow regulatory T cells or BM Tregs are characterized by the cell membrane signature CD4+ CD25+ (some prefer to call it "bright") FOXP3+. These figures and numbers are like a barcode for this kind of cell type that is found within the lymphocyte population of cells in the BM. The CD4+ marker tells us that they are T cells. It is not important to know the details of what molecules the barcode stand for. The important point is the unique function that these BM Tregs have on the immune system. These cells are very specific suppressors of host anti-cancer immunity. In newly diagnosed patients with MM, the BM contains a large percentage of Tregs. With successful treatment, the percentage of BM Tregs is expected to decrease. However, for patients with progressive disease, the percentage of BM Tregs is expected to increase.

Using an assay call indirect immunofluorescence flow cytometric analysis or immunophenotyping, BM Tregs were enumerated in this patient before and after he achieved complete remission (CR) with the "dtZ" regimen (Fig. 6.21). This patient had a very brisk response to "dtZ" and achieved CR after only three cycles of "dtZ." The BM examination was performed after he achieved CR and ISS "Stage Zero" (see below); and when the ANC, absolute lymphocyte counts, normal IgG, IgA and IgM levels were all normal. The second quadrant contains the CD4+ CD25+ Treg population of cells. A window is drawn to focus on the Tregs. (FOXP3 stains were not routinely performed by this lab. In any case, the majority of the CD4+ CD25+ cell population is also usually

136 *Towards Individualized Therapy for Multiple Myeloma*

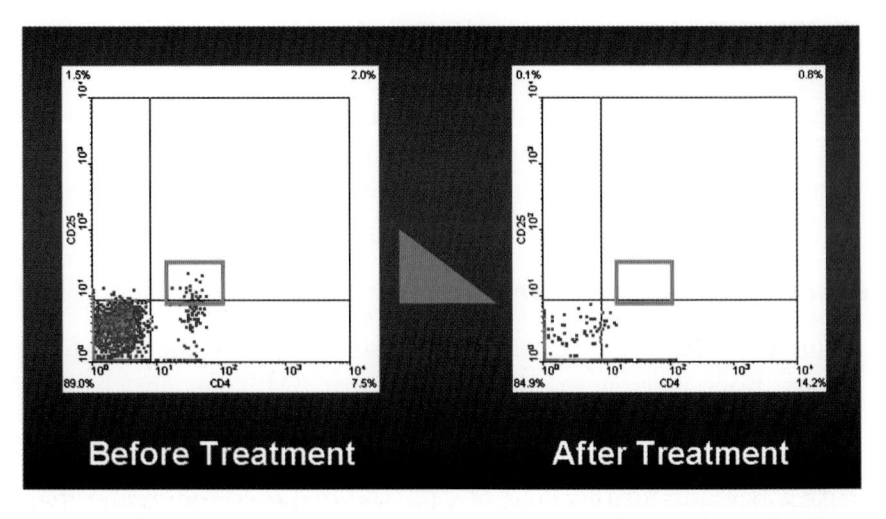

Fig. 6.21. Decreased BM Tregs in a patient successfully treated with "dtZ".

FOXP3+.) It is not difficult to see that there is a near total absence of Tregs in the BM after successful treatment with "dtZ." The data is fully consistent with the abrogation of immunosuppression in the BM and return of host anti-tumor immunity. It is possible that this patient could achieve a highly-durable remission.

In the opposite scenario, this is a patient who did not respond to "dtZ" (Fig. 6.22). At the time of reassessment, her ANC, normal Igs and absolute lymphocyte count were all below normal. In other words, her immunity was suppressed in line with the increased BM Tregs after treatment.

We analyzed the percentage change in BM Tregs in 15 patients before and after treatment with six cycles of "dtZ." Patients were assessed for their clinical response to treatment using established (Blade's) criteria — CR, PR, minimal response (MR) and progressive disease (PD). As can be seen in Fig. 6.23, the percentage change in BM Tregs was a perfect correlation with the clinical response to treatment. These data confirmed that BM Tregs were a good parameter to use in assessing a patient's response to anti-MM treatment. Moreover, because BM Tregs are an immunological marker,

Multiple Myeloma 137

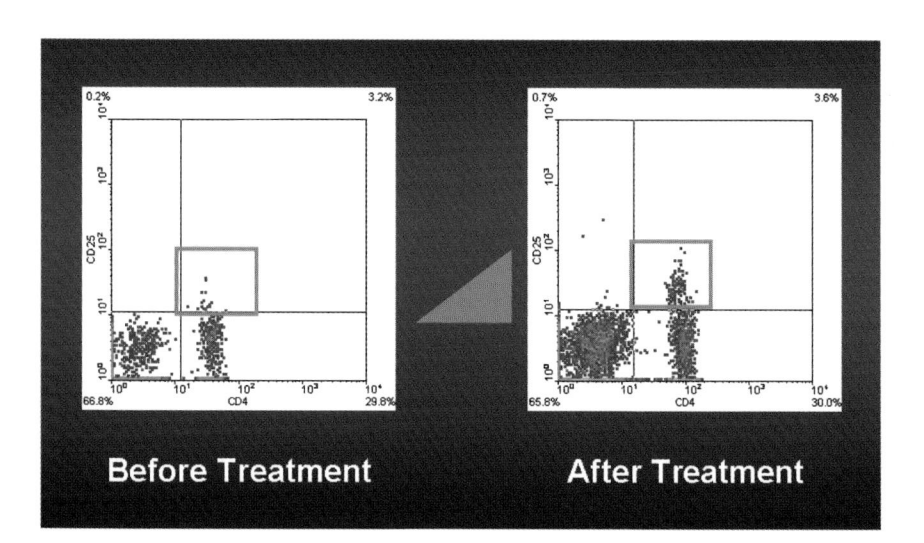

Fig. 6.22. Increased BM Tregs in a patient with progressive disease after "dtZ".

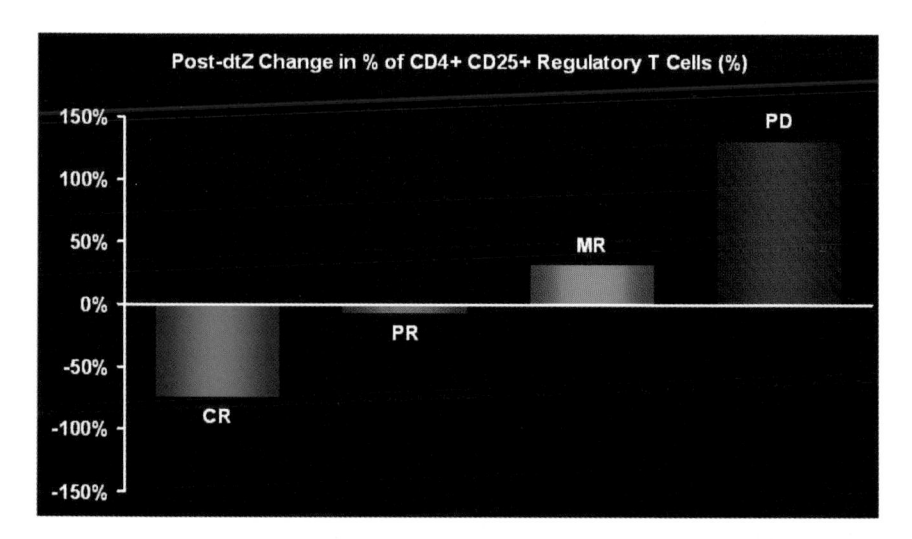

Fig. 6.23. Percentage of BM Tregs correlates with depth of response in patients treated with "dtZ".

138 *Towards Individualized Therapy for Multiple Myeloma*

this data strongly supports the notion that successful treatment using individualized targeted therapy with the "dtZ" regimen was associated with restitution of host anti-MM immunity. Hence, it would not be unreasonable to expect patients who achieve low BM Tregs and clinical CR to benefit from a more durable remission.

Deciding Therapy by Immunological Profiling

I had previously provided the ISS staging system, which has three stages; I, II and III (Table 2.5, p.). In deciding which patients to wean off treatment, I frequently use the concept of ISS "Stage Zero" (Table 6.13). To attain ISS "Stage Zero," patients must have totally normal albumin and B2M levels. There is an overlap between ISS stage I and "Stage Zero," i.e. some patients with ISS stage I can be considered as "Stage Zero." Please note that "Stage Zero" is not part of the ISS staging system, it is a way of helping us to individualize treatment for the patient.

Weaning off Step 1 — Lightening Treatment

There are basically two checkpoints or steps in weaning off patients from intensive therapy. The goal of Step 1 is to lighten treatment to allow recovery of the immune system. This should be done only when tumor burden is low, i.e. ISS "Stage Zero." Patients with ISS "Stage Zero" may still have a residual M-band

Table 6.13.   The Concept of "Stage Zero"

ISS Stage	Albumin (g/L)	B2M (mg/L)
0	≥ 37	≤ 2.0
I	≥ 35	≤ 3.5
II	< 35	3.5 to 5.5
III	< 35	> 5.5

and are analogous to having very good partial response (VGPR) or an MGUS-like state.

Weaning off Step 2 — Maintenance Therapy

The goal of Step 2 is to convert treatment to a monotherapy maintenance regimen that can be tolerated for an extended period of time. In other words, patients are more or less going to be on their own with a little help from their doctors. The patients must be in ISS "Stage Zero" and have full recovery of the ANC, normal IgG, IgA and IgM levels as well as normal lymphocyte counts. A BM examination demonstrates low BM Treg levels provide added confidence to commence maintenance therapy.

Chapter 7

CURRENT TREATMENT

"Individualized Therapy...more than just the evidence."

The key subparameters that relate to currently-available therapies are:

- Experiential medicine
- Experimental medicine
- Evidence-based medicine
- Execution/application of treatments

This may be a difficult topic for some of us to understand, i.e. the group dynamics that govern experiential, experimental, evidence-based and applied medicine (Fig. 7.1), because the boundaries are not so clear to the unfamiliar. In order not to confuse you further, I will use our experiences in the development of the "dtZ" regimen as an example of how one can individualize therapy using anti-MM drugs which are currently available. But I hope that you agree that it makes no sense for me to provide a list of all the therapeutic possibilities available today and to discuss their effectiveness, either alone or in combination. To do this would be akin to writing an entire encyclopedia, which will probably become obsolete as soon as I finish. I would consider it more worthwhile to do a case study and in the course understand the processes that are involved in individualizing treatment for patients with MM.

140

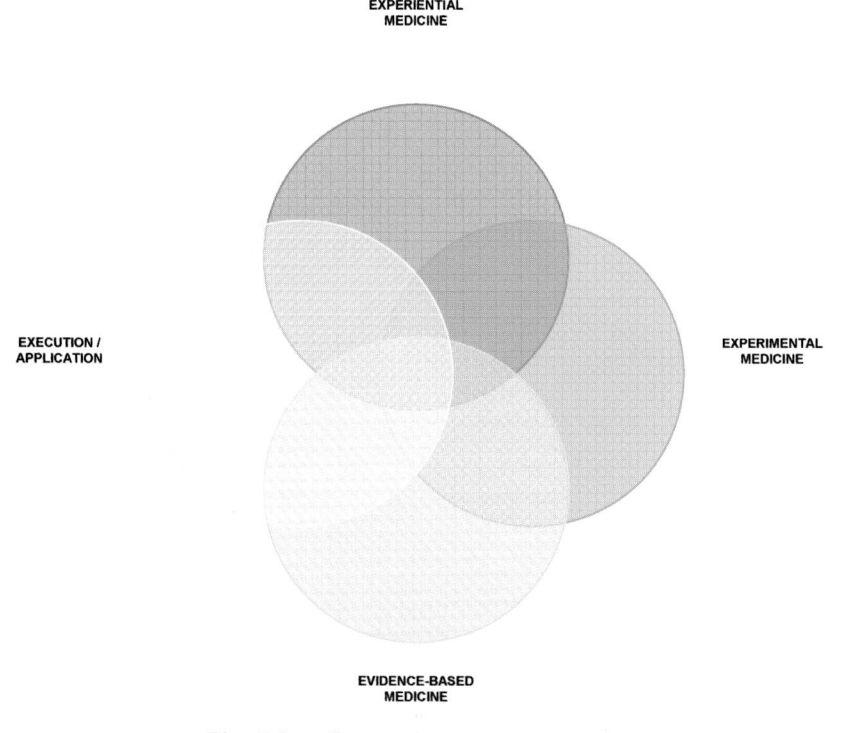

Fig. 7.1. Current treatment parameters.

Today, we have what some would call a "good" problem to have, i.e. the luxury of having more compounds than we can possibly swatch around. And in all honesty, even if we were able to put the bulk of these through clinical trials, we would not have figured them out before newer compounds were discovered. We are indeed spoilt for choice, and that is not an understatement. But this sets the stage up for us to really work some magic in individualizing treatments for patients. Because we only have basic guidelines to devise regimens that work, we rely greatly on logical reasoning and careful selection of laboratory data that are related to the drugs we are using. With these in the background, let's now look more closely at the "making of dtZ." In particular, I would like you to focus on the logic and group dynamics that revolve around the patient, his disease and the drugs that are being used as these will help you better understand what individualizing therapy for patients means. Please be mindful that "dtZ" is just one of the many ways to individualize therapy in MM; there are many other ways of doing the same thing. In fact, I am hoping that in the future you will put on your thinking caps and devise other versions of individualized therapy of your own that you will one day put into clinical practice. If you can do this, I would feel that I have made the difference in your patients' lives.

Experiential Medicine

The vision of the "dtZ" project was to find a treatment regimen that was easily customizable for patients with MM. It was a deliberate attempt to individualize therapy. In its mission, four fundamental issues were addressed:

- The regimen should be minimal so that individualization would be simple. There should be no more than three or four drugs.
- The immune system should be preserved. In other words, cytotoxic drugs would be avoided at all costs. C ə B — cyto toxic
- Management of MM bone disease should be foremost; in particular the elimination of OCs and the blockade of the "Monocyte Loop."
- Patients must feel comfortable throughout treatment so that they gain confidence with the regimen. Side effects must be kept to a minimum and tolerance to therapy should be built up.

In the initial stages, the concept of experience (experiential medicine) was applied. Three non-cytotoxic drugs — dexamethasone (d), thalidomide (t) and zoledronic acid (Z) — were selected. Of these, dexamethasone was the oldest and the one with the best experiences. Hence, dexamethasone formed the backbone of therapy. By contrast, thalidomide and zoledronic acid were relatively new agents at that time and there was somewhat limited clinical experience. Accordingly, I had to turn to the gurus of MM. My personal communications with leading experts in MM in the world, especially Professor Kenneth Anderson, provided tremendous amount of insight into the design of the backbone of the regimen, i.e. pulsed dexamethasone. Specifically, a 3-weekly cycle in which dexamethasone was given in weekly pulses was recommended. This provided us immediately with the golden opportunity to use high dose rate zoledronic acid 3-weekly. As discussed in the chapters above, our initial experiences with zoledronic acid, as well as close scrutiny of published literature at that time supported this approach. So now we had a 3-weekly regimen of dexamethasone and zoledronic acid (Fig. 7.2), and just the doses to fit in. The dose of zoledronic acid was easiest. It was provided as a 4.0 mg vial and at 3-weekly dosing would on average provide an EQmg/ month of ~6.0. This I considered optimal.

However, dosing of dexamethasone despite its long history was tricky. It might surprise you that after nearly two to three decades of dexamethasone use in MM, no one really knows the optimal dose of dexamethasone to use. It was common knowledge that dexamethasone was the most active agent in combination chemotherapy protocols like VAD, but the optimal dose of dexamethasone was elusive. In VAD, the dose of dexamethasone was quite high, ~480 mg/month. A gentler version of VAD (which I like to call "VAD-lite") from the Mayo Clinic in Minnesota was

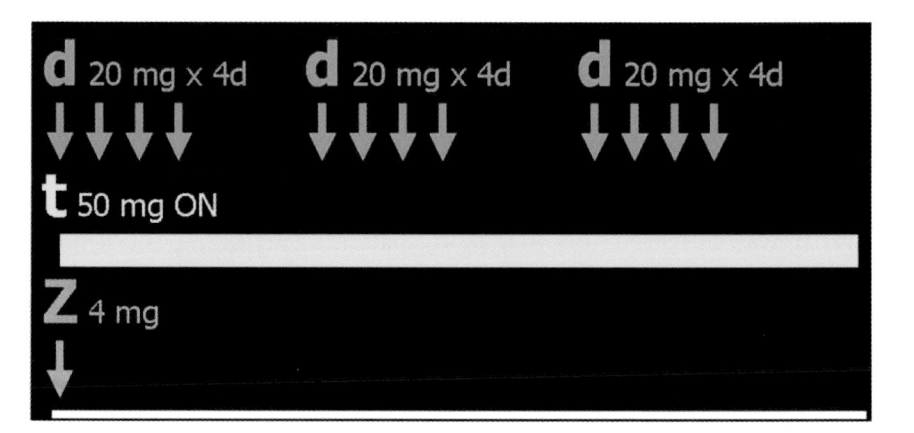

Fig. 7.2. The "dtZ" regimen.

~320 mg/month. This was associated with a better patient tolerance and side effects profile. So I chose to give 320 mg/month, which was in line with our mission statement, i.e. to use the lowest recommended doses of dexamethasone and thalidomide. I felt that complex regimens would confuse patients, nurses and doctors, and invite more problems than necessary. Hence, quite arbitrarily I decided to introduce a simple weekly dosing schedule for dexamethasone so that patients could get these smaller doses, then have some time off to recover and then start again. This regimen would then be repeated monotonously as part of the patient's daily treatment routine until the patient became so used to it that they would not forget taking their medicine. By simple mathematics, dexamethasone was given 320 mg a month, or 80 mg a week, or 20 mg per day for four days every week. Patients then had three days to rest before starting over again (Fig. 7.2). In other words, patients were "educated" to maintain a routine of "four days on and three days off" every week.

Finally, it came to fitting thalidomide into the regimen. To do this, I actually turned the equation on its head. You see, at that point of time, thalidomide was just starting to make waves in the MM scene; and everyone was trying to devise regimens that included thalidomide; e.g. the very famous "Thal-Dex" regimen. In actual fact, "dtZ" is basically a variant "Thal-Dex" regimen. The difference between "dtZ" and the other "Thal-Dex" regimens was that thalidomide was the backbone of the traditional "Thal-Dex" regimen, and everything else was fashioned around it. In "dtZ," dexamethasone plus zoledronic acid was backbone and thalidomide was fashioned around it. This came about because of the clinical experience with the index patient I presented earlier (Fig. 6.19). What was observed was that many patients (including the index patient) could not tolerate regular doses of thalidomide. Not surprising because the rate of major toxicities related to regular dose "Thal-Dex" was not much different from combination chemotherapy regimens like VAD. In other words, regular dose "Thal-Dex" was not an innocuous regimen; it was fairly toxic. Hence, using my observations/experiences with thalidomide, I layered thalidomide over the dexamethasone-zoledronic acid backbone slowly and carefully to find the optimal dose of thalidomide. I cannot over-emphasize the importance of experiential medicine at this stage of development of the "dtZ" regimen. It was through observation and experience that permitted us to individualize thalidomide to doses that were both effective as well as tolerable. So the rules for using thalidomide unfolded before us:

- Thalidomide takes time to start; its action was not immediate.
- Even tiny doses (e.g. 50 mg weekly) appeared to have some effect.
- The maximum tolerable dose before any side effects (including minor side effects) occurred was between 50 mg and 100 mg a day.
- Pulsing thalidomide was not a good thing to do; it had to be given continuously and tailed-off gradually.

Our experience suggested that individualized low-dose thalido-mide was ~50 mg daily, and this became the basic dose for the "dtZ" regimen (Fig. 7.2). Feedback from patients who used the regimen was highly favorable. Most felt that it was well-tolerated and remarkably easy to follow. Certain rules for dose adjustments were thrown in later on to tweak the regimen further. But overall, the clinical experience was extremely rewarding. So, it was time to test it out.

Experimental Medicine

I had earlier presented this graph of the expected results of conventional therapies for newly-diagnosed patients with MM (Fig. 4.6). I have now updated it with the inclusion of the data from 26 patients with relapsed and refractory MM (but not untreated MM) who were given the "dtZ" regimen (Fig. 7.3, red line).[67-70] After following the cohort for four to six years, you can easily see from the graphs that these patients behaved quite differently from conventionally-treated patients. At about 28 months,

146   *Towards Individualized Therapy for Multiple Myeloma*

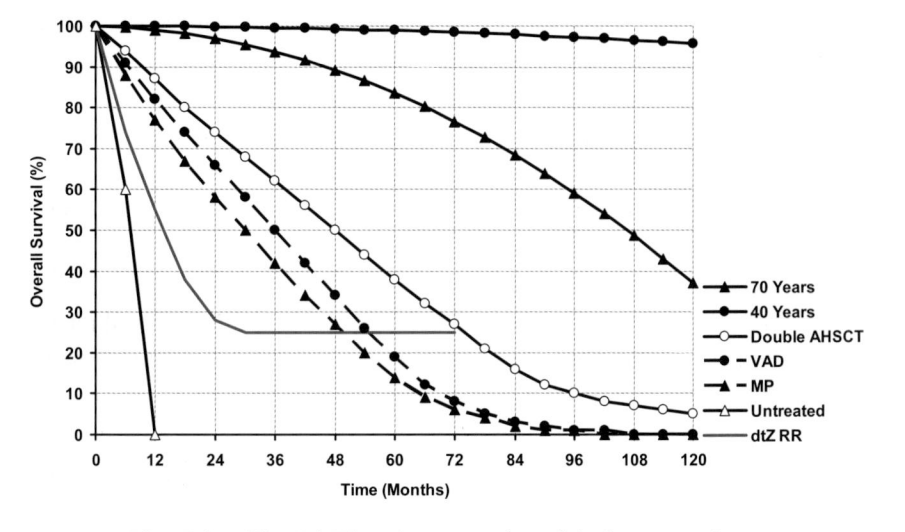

Fig. 7.3.   The "dtZ" regimen — relapsed/refractory patients.

there appeared to be an inflexion point and patients who survived till then appeared to be "cured." What is not shown in this small but highly provocative group of patients is that 7 of the 26 patients had achieved VGPR, nCR or CR. These seven patients then went on to become long-term survivors, suggesting that very good depth of response (i.e. VGPR, nCR or CR) was critical for durability of response. By contrast 19 of 26 patients who failed to achieve VGPR, nCR or CR did poorly and died before 28 months from the time of starting treatment. This data concurs totally with the observations of other researchers; that patients who achieved the low tumor burden states (i.e. VGPR or better) went on to have the best responses. The fact that some patients achieved nCR and CR is also a clear endorsement of the effectiveness of a seemingly minimal or light regimen. Indeed, less seemed to be more. In aggregate, we now had the pilot experimental results to formally test the "dtZ" regimen in a formal clinical trial. This is important because designing any clinical trial requires a certain amount of basic experimental (pilot study) information. Ironically, whereas so much effort was spent to individualize therapy and devise a regimen that catered to the patient, a formal clinical trial would now

Current Treatment   147

prevent any further attempt at individualization until the trial was over. Such, such irony — the bane of medical evidence!

Evidence-based Medicine (EBM)

Whilst I will not be able to exhibit study data because it is embargoed for scientific publication, I will nonetheless "simulate" the data with a subset of 22 patients that used the "dtZ" regimen as their first line of treatment, but outside the setting of a clinical trial. This data should of course be considered as only preliminary, as it is neither unedited nor unverified. Its purpose is only for discussion. When patients with newly-diagnosed MM were now given the "dtZ" regimen instead of conventional therapy in the setting of a formal clinical trial, the first observation that was made was that the RRs were very high. The expected RRs for conventional chemotherapy is about 50–55% and for tandem AHSCT is about 70–75%. The observed RR for "dtZ" was greater than 80%. As can be seen in Fig. 7.4 (blue line), the survival curves clearly deviate

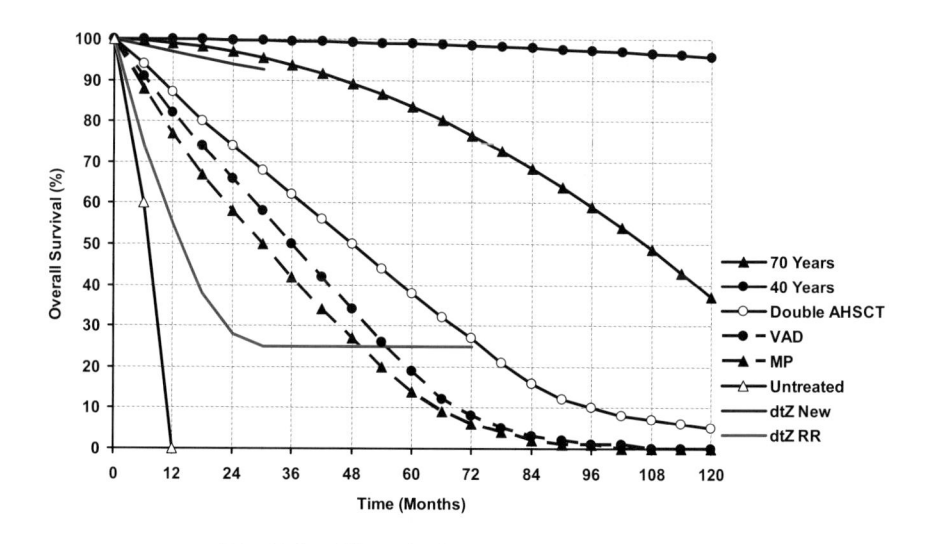

Fig. 7.4. The "dtZ" regimen — new patients.

148   *Towards Individualized Therapy for Multiple Myeloma*

from the conventional trends for a variety of representative therapies. In fact, survival data for both relaspsed/refractory (Fig. 20C red line) as well as newly-diagnosed (Fig. 20C blue line) MM patients given "dtZ" demonstrate significantly longer-term survival than all other forms of therapy. Collectively, both experience and now experiment have provided clear evidence that individualization of therapy for patients with MM is not only possible, it is highly-efficacious and desirable.

Execution/Application

The stage is now set for execution or application of this data into the real world setting. Actually, moving forward, there are two directions that can be pursued:

Clinical Application

To test if patients who received individualized targeted therapies can do even better than those in the clinical trial. Importantly, these patients now included patients who would have been excluded form the clinical trial because they would have failed the eligibility criteria. Patients are firstly treated *ad lib* with an individualized regimen that is both superior and safe. This treatment is tweaked further for maximal optimization. We must always be aware and exercise flexibility when treating patients with terminal diseases like cancer. Every effort should be made to achieve the best outcome. Most importantly, patients should not be deprived of effective treatment at the expense of bureaucratic restrictions.

Further Clinical Testing

It is customary for clinical trials that have shown efficacy (so-called Phase II studies) to be tested on a larger group of patients. This is to see if there are biases that could have arisen because of the relatively small size of Phase II studies that would now become more obvious when more statistical data is obtained. These Phase III studies also have the feature of pitting one regimen against another in an effort to further establish the superiority of a regimen. Even newer and hopefully more useful data is generated in Phase III studies. Unfortunately, the return to a clinical trial is again restrictive when the aim is the pursuit of individualization. But at this stage, it is a test on an already individualized regimen; not quite as bad as the Phase II study when the regimen had not undergone much individualization.

Chapter **8**

FUTURE OPPORTUNITIES

"Manage your expectations well."

The key subparameters that relate to future opportunities for a patient are:

- Academic sponsors
- Pharmaceutical sponsors
- Commercial sponsors
- Health regulators.

This section is probably best written as a single group, rather than individually, because of the similarities in the roles of these agencies in fostering individualization of therapy for MM. Accordingly, the weaknesses of a particular agency may be rescued by the strength of another. There will probably be too many policy differences to be discussed, which like the available choices of drugs that can be used to treat MM, are better left out of the discussion so as not to delve too much in minutiae at the expense of overriding principles. The bottom line is, in order for individualization to succeed, all agencies must be considered equally important and must be encouraged to work together in the most creative fashion towards a common goal, i.e. improved healthcare. Easier said than done because it is unrealistic to expect the world to be

150

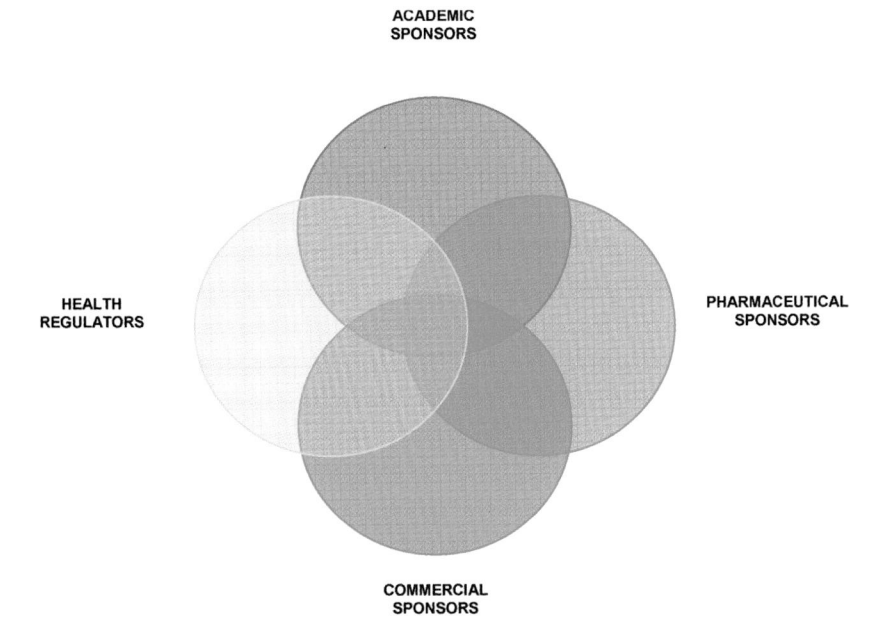

Fig. 8.1. Future opportunities parameters.

perfect. Perhaps 80% is a good goal to have. In other words, if there is synergy for 80% of the time, we will have a chance to move forward. For the rough edges in the remaining 20%, the constant question will be to compete or to collaborate. Without a doubt, egos and idiosyncrasies will get in the way; but with determination, vision and a lot of creativity, there are bound to be successes. The finesse will be finding the person with the X-factor and then all the pieces of the jigsaw puzzle will fall into place. Again, I will use the "dtZ" regimen to discuss how the remaining four parameters (Fig. 8.1) affect our opportunities for individualized therapy for MM in the future.

Academic Sponsors

I think the best way to approach the discussion is to look at the system constraints. It is fairly easy to understand the vision and mission statements of various healthcare agencies, but the crux of the matter is; what are the constraints in their different systems that will make this treatment fail or fail to even enter the market. This is not a fault-finding exercise, but more of a reality check. This reality check is very important because it helps us manage our expectations better. So where are the system constraints in academia that will make it more difficult for us to find newer therapies for MM patients? Without sounding like a wet blanket, there are essentially three major system constraints:

- Use of public funds
- Inflexibility of systematic peer review
- Lack of true talent in public institutions.

Use of Public Funds

Public academic bodies are funded by public funds — a no-brainer, we can all understand that. There is a limit to the funds that are available. The pie must be shared equally to protect public interest. There must be rules on how to share the money. Every man in the street is a stakeholder in these funds and public academic bodies must protect his interests. After all, it is his money we are using to develop new therapies for patients with MM. Because he is a stakeholder, he is allowed to put some brakes on the system, and he is in a sense allowed to pull the plug if things go wrong. This is bureaucracy but a necessity for things to carry on in an orderly fashion.

Inflexibility of Systematic Peer Review

What happens when we try to tap on public funds for research? This involves the processes by which research projects are "tendered" for by wannabe researchers. This tendering system is a typical feature of public service departments. There is nothing wrong with doing this, except that it puts weights on the ankles of researchers, especially the young and talented who are just starting out. The process is, let's face it, slow. Moreover, it's a catch-22 for the virgins, "no data, no funds" and "no funds, no data." Of course there are so-called incubator programs to nurture these wannabe researchers but these are often shrouded by other layers of peer review. In an effort to circumvent some of the obstacles and jump start the engine, hybrid systems where some of the red tape has been cut, whilst others have been streamlined, have been creatively crafted by teams of more experienced persons. These usually take a toll on the sense of fair play as some level of "oiling" is usually required to get the engines warmed up. My own experience is that they have been met with variable and/or sporadic successes.

Lack of True Talent in Public Institutions

This is where I might sound somewhat cynical, and believe me, I have tried my level best to stay out of cynicism. But let's face it, this is a real problem in public institutions. In this less than ideal situation, the best and smartest (rats) are the first to "abandon" ship. Talented individuals leave the public service for whatever reason. And the public service is left with... There is a limit to what a deeply bureaucratic system can provide for the most talented of individuals. At a certain point, something's gotta give and these persons will without much hesitation leave for greener pastures. This has been called the "push factor." But it is not as though private academic institutions are not lacking talented individuals. They also have a talent lack but of a different nature. In the private sector, because talent is still relatively scarce, these chaps get headhunted by other private institutions. You can call this the "pull factor." Yes, the private sector will have talent skewed in its favor, but this talent is diluted. Hence, if you had to wager where the future of better and more innovative individualized treatments lies, my last dollar will be in private academia; because that's where most of the talented researchers are.

In the development of the "dtZ" regimen, academic research provided about 30% of the resources needed to accomplish the project. These were mainly human capital, i.e. the patients who

154 *Towards Individualized Therapy for Multiple Myeloma*

attended the clinics in the public hospitals. They played a critical role to the development of the regimen that was individualized to their needs. Despite what I had written above, I would not discount the importance of academic sponsorship. The point to emphasize is there is a distinct system limit that cannot be overcome by any means within that system. For the future of MM therapy, one has to look beyond academic sponsors.

Pharmaceutical Sponsors

In my opinion, these are the most important players in the quest for future MM treatments and renewed hope for patients with MM. Pharmaceutical sponsors who are capable of bringing in new products and ideas to test will certainly light up the life of both doctors and patients. In "dtZ's" development, pharmaceutical sponsors supported 50% of the research and development (R&D). Without a doubt, pharmaceutical sponsors are critical to the success of forward-moving individualized therapies. If you wanted any advice from me as to who to engage when trying to develop an individualized regimen for any disease, it would be the pharmaceutical companies. However, they have one very distinct thorn in the flesh — bias. You cannot remove this from the equation. Every time you talk about their new drug, someone will think you are biased. But what company is going to promote its competitor's product? You would be totally naïve to think that the pharmaceutical company will not be thinking of marketing the compound from Day 1. Is there a way out of this?

Actually, there is but it is not perfect. The answer is what we call an "Investigator-Initiated Trial" or IIT. In the setting of an IIT, the academic investigator (whether public or private academia) is given permission by the pharmaceutical company to pursue his research idea at the expense of the pharmaceutical company. Sounds like a fairy tale. Let me elaborate. There is no free lunch; research must of course be approved by the pharmaceutical company. The key to success is synergy. Develop a healthy investigator-company relationship in the setting of the IIT. When the investigator-company relationship is set up in this format, the company seemingly relinquishes its marketing intention and the investigator becomes the "sponsor." The issue is trust. Very few pharmaceutical companies trust their investigators enough to give them this (albeit limited) "liberty" to do what they want. But believe me, there are numerous opportunities to have a common intent where the investigator-company relationship can flourish. Sincere cooperativeness is much to be applauded for. It is with this genuineness of intent and trust that made the difference to "dtZ." You see, "dtZ" was developed as an IIT. There was almost perfect synergy between the academic institutions (public and private) and the pharmaceutical company. The investigator (myself) was given the freedom to fashion an individualized regimen for MM patients using the compound from the company in a "win-win" format. And in the end, it was win-win-win for patient, doctor and company. Without even thinking twice about it, I would fully encourage wannabe researchers to go down the IIT alley.

Commercial Sponsors

These are an added resource in two scenarios:

- Programs that are struggling to succeed
- Programs that have very high potential that need a leg up

Since "dtZ" was neither, our involvement with commercial sponsors was 0%. I will not discuss too much about commercial sponsors except to say that the engagement of this category of sponsors is more risky than the others. Yes, the problem here is commercial risk. As someone in the industry once told me, "You have to be prepared to lose your shirt and pants when you are working with these types of resources." My own personal view is that in the medical field, where there is already a great amount of risk, it is not fair to "gamble" using patients as chips. Some level of safety must always be built in when handling lives. Moreover, the integrity of the investigator is a virtue that needs to be protected constantly. True academia may not provide the flexibility and speed of commercial sponsorship; but the higher stakes and unpredictability of return on investment in healthcare make uncharted waters particularly hazardous for the inexperienced. The bottom line is, go at your own risk. And if you are not experienced, prepare to fail.

Health Regulators

Finally, the all-important health regulators. Unlike other diseases, cancer is considered to be a terminal disease where patients' rights are fundamentally upheld. Fortunately most health regulators remain sympathetic to patients and there is little to fault the patient when life-or-death decisions are debated. The overriding principal in the development of logical and safe anti-cancer therapies is the hope that these treatments will prolong life. Longevity is the gold standard of effective treatment. In countries with good governments and where healthcare is managed well, there should not be any problems with health regulators. They safeguard the interests of the patient above all else. The problem is the proliferation of wannabe health regulators who conjure up their own regulations, i.e. people who do not have any authority but who freely advise according to their own perceptions of the state of affairs. Surprisingly, it is rather easy to find opinionated persons who freely advise on matters that are not within their jurisdiction. And I will be the first to admit that there are many of these in the medical profession. In "dtZ" we worked with health regulators about 20% of the time. We received advice from almost everybody, so be careful.

Chapter **9**

CONCLUDING REMARKS

"Individualized therapy is for every MM patient because they are special and deserve to be treated as individuals."

Look first at your patient from a bird's eye view. Consider him/her as an individual. Consider that what you have decided to treat him/her with will NOT work in the way you intended it. Consider that you will need to change the regimen. Make changes to treatment that work towards specific goals that are associated with logical outcomes; e.g. lowering AMCO levels. Rather than accept age-old concepts, think out of the box. Keep molding treatment until it fits him/her. Learn to juggle all 20 parameters at the same time, understand the group dynamics. Step back and look again…your patient has now become a special individual. Motivate your patient and see the magic of individualized therapy unfold…

ABBREVIATIONS

Ab	Antibody
ADL	Activities of daily living
AHSCT	Autologous hemopoietic stem cell transplantation
AMCO	Absolute monocyte count
AMM	Asymptomatic multiple myeloma
ANC	Absolute neutrophil count
B2M	Beta-2-microglobulin
BCG	Bacillus Calmet-Guerin
BM	Bone marrow
BMD	Bone mineral density
BMSC	Bone marrow stromal cell
BSA	Body surface area
CBC	Complete blood count
CD40L	CD40 ligand
CMV	Cytomegalovirus
CR	Complete response
CRP	C-reactive protein
CS	Catalytic subunit
CT scan	Computer tomographic scan
DEXA scan	(DXA scan) Dual-emission X-ray absoptiometric scan
DNA-PK	DNA protein kinase
DSBR	DNA double-strand break repair
dtZ	Dexamethasone, thalidomide and zoledronic acid
EBM	Evidence-based medicine

159

ECM	Extracellular matrix
EMM	Early multiple myeloma
FBC	Full blood count
G-CSF	Granulocyte colony-stimulating factor
GEP	Gene expression profiling
GOF	Gain of function
GP	General practitioner
Hb	Hemoglobin
HBV	Hepatitis B virus
HPV	Human papillomavirus
HR	Homologous recombination
iCSR	Isotype class switch recombination
ICU	Intensive care unit
IF	Immunofixation
Ig	Immunoglobulin
IgA	Immunoglobulin class A
IgD	Immunoglobulin class D
IgE	Immunoglobulin class E
IgG	Immunoglobulin class G
IgH	Immunoglobulin heavy chain
IgM	Immunoglobulin class M
IIS	Investigator-initiated study
IIT	Investigator-initiated trial
IL-4	Interleukin-4
IL-6	Interleukin-6
ISS	International staging system
LC	Light chain
LDH	Lactate dehydrogenase
LOF	Loss of function
LP	Lumbar puncture
mAb	Monoclonal antibody
MAHA	Mouse antihuman antibodies
MDS	Myelodysplastic syndrome
MGUS	Monoclonal gammopathy of undetermined significance
MM	Multiple myeloma

MP	Melphalan and prednisolone
MPD	Myeloproliferative disorder
MR	Minimal response
MRI scan	Magnetic resonance imaging scan
NCCN	National Cancer Care Network
nCR	Near complete response
NHEJ	Non-homologous end-joining
OB	Osteoblast
OC	Osteoclast
ONJ	Osteonecrosis of the jaw
PB	Peripheral blood
PCL	Plasma cell leukemia
PD	Progressive disease
PET scan	Positron emission technology scan
PNY	Peripheral neuropathy
pOC	Precursor osteoclast
POEMS	Polyradiculopathy, organomegaly, endocrinopathy, M-protein and skin changes
PR	Partial response
Pred	Prednisolone
QoL	Quality of life
R&D	Research and development
SARS	Severe acute respiratory syndrome
SCID	Severe combined immunodeficiency
SD	Standard deviation
SRE	Skeletal related event
Treg	Regulatory T cells
TSA	Tumor-specific antigen
VAD	Vincristine, adriamycin and dexamethasone
VGPR	Very good partial response

GLOSSARY

Adenoma	Tumor masses that contain glandular tissue.
Anemia	The clinical state of having lower than normal red blood cell levels or counts.
Angiogenesis	The process of blood vessel formation.
Anergy	Lack of responsiveness, usually of T lymphocytes towards a specific stimulus.
Antibody	Proteins that are produced by special cells of the immune system called plasma cells. Antibodies are protective to our bodies, they help to fight germs and foreign substances.
Apheresis	The process by which blood cells are selected and harvested from a living person using centrifuge-like machine that is attached to the person's circulatory system.
Apoptosis	Programmed cell death. All cells are programmed to die unless they become immortalized, e.g. by cancer causing processes.
Applied research	This refers to research for the creation of products (e.g. drugs and devices) that can be used for clinical treatment.
B cells/ lymphocytes	Cells of the immune system that eventually produce antibodies.
Basic research	This refers to very fundamental research studies performed usually in a laboratory.

Benign	Not malicious; not cancer.
Bone marrow	The blood-forming organ that is present inside the bones of the skeleton.
Bone mineral density	The relative density of bone associated with its calcium content.
Bone scan	A radioactive body scan in which the detecting substance (also called a tracer) is a radioactive isotope which emits radioactive rays that can be detected by photographic film.
Bronchiectasis	A chronic lung condition caused by permanent damage to the air passages of the lungs such that secretions collect like pools in the lung tissue. Such pools of secretions are easily infected by germs and extremely difficult to remove.
Cell culture	Technique of growing living cells outside the body in an incubator.
Cell lines	Explanted cells have been kept in continuous cell culture generation after generation.
Chemotherapy	Treatment of cancer using toxic chemicals (called cytotoxic drugs) that kill cancer cells as well as normal cells.
Chromosome	The DNA polymer is like a very long string of beads which carry the genetic code. This DNA polymer folded and coiled up many, many times over into a structure known as a chromosome. Every human cell has 46 chromosomes.
Chromosomal translocation	When a part of a chromosome gets transferred or relocated to another chromosome by some abnormal genetic event.
Colonoscopy	Examination of the large intestine (colon and rectum) using a fiberoptic camera device called a colonoscope.
CT scan	Sophisticated X-ray-based body scan where computer algorithms are used to piece together

	image information from multiple serial layers of X-rays.
"CRAB"	The diagnostic clinical acronym of MM which stands for: hyperCalcemia, Renal failure, Anemia and Bone pain/disease.
DEXA/DXA scan	Soft X-ray body scan of certain parts of the skeleton, e.g. the spine or the hips, that is used to determine the relative density of the bones associated with its calcium content.
Dysregulation	Disruption of normal regulation.
Evidence-based medicine	The practice of medicine based on published and peer-reviewed data, particularly those from human clinical trials.
Explant	To remove from the original host. In the case of cancer, this refers to tissue that has been removed from the original tumor mass in the body.
Extracellular matrix	Non-cellular substances (like glue) that are found outside cells in the microenvironment.
Fibroblasts	Soft tissue cells that provide a support function.
Full skeletal survey	Plan X-ray scan of the entire body looking especially at the skeletal structure.
Gastroscopy	Examination of the gullet (esophagus), stomach and upper portion of the small intestine (duodenum) using a fiberoptic camera device called a gastroscope.
Gene	The part of the DNA genetic code that is active in producing proteins for cellular processes.
Gene deletion	When a part of the DNA genetic code is removed or missing.
Gene expression profiling	The profile (as a snapshot in time) of the genetic events can be analyzed for a single cell today. The genes that are expressed and so profiled can be tracked over time by analyzing another cell at a later point in time, creating a "story" of genetic events in e.g. a cancer.

Gene microarray analysis	A highly sophisticated gene analysis method that surveys literally thousands of genes at the same time. The method uses a microscope slide on which are "printed" in a tiny array of dots genes of interest for that analysis.
Gene mutation	When part of the DNA genetic code is changed.
Glomeruli	Small mesh-like structures in the kidneys where water and water-soluble substances filter through from the blood stream into the renal tubules (see below) in process of urine formation.
Glucocorticoid	A steroid-like drug.
Host tumor immuno-surveillance	The protective function of the immune system to police the body for cancer cells and to get rid of them before cancer develops.
Hypercalcemia	The clinical state of having higher than normal levels calcium in the blood.
Hyperdiploidy	Having more chromosomes (see above) than normal.
Hypocalcemia	The clinical state of having lower than normal levels of calcium in the blood.
Hypodiploidy	Having fewer chromosomes (see above) than normal.
Ileus	A clinical state of paralysis of the intestines. In other words, the intestines are unable to perform their normal function to move digested food towards the anus for excretion.
Immune system	The defense system of the body that protects us from germs and other foreign substances. It is known for its healing properties. The immune system is also thought to protect the body against cancer; to be able to perform surveillance for cancer cells in the body and to literally kill the cancer cells.

Immuno-compromise	Weakening of the immune system to a point that there is some danger of breaching by foreign invaders.
Immunocytes	Cells of the immune system
Immunoglobulin	A more technical name for antibody (see above). There are five classes of immunoglobulins or Igs — IgA, IgD, IgE, IgG and IgM.
Immunoglobulin heavy chains	Immunoglobulins are made up of two heavy chains and two light chains. The heavy chain varieties are: α, δ, ϵ, γ and μ.
Immunoglobulin light chains	Immunoglobulins are made up of two heavy chains and two light chains. The light chain varieties are: κ and λ.
Immunoparesis	Weakening of the immune system.
Immuno-phenotyping	Also called indirect immunofluorescence flow cytometric analysis, is the analysis of the identity of cells using markers that are expressed on the surface of the cell membrane.
Immuno-protection	Protection of the body by the immune system.
Immuno-suppression	Weakening of the immune system by an external agent, e.g. steroid drugs.
Induction therapy	Treatment that is first introduced to control the cancer.
Infarction	Death of tissues and/or organs of the body by cessation of blood supply.
Inflexion point	A point in a graph where the trend of the graph makes a sharp turn, so much so as to suggest that there is a very significant change in the behavior of that parameter.
Inotropes	Drugs that help to improve the contractions of the heart and thereby improve (low) blood pressure states.
International Staging System	This is the most current prognostic risk stratification system used in MM.

Intravenous	Injection directly into the vein.
Karyotype	The quality of the set of chromosomes present in a cell.
Ligand	A substance that attaches to a cell receptor that can produce a signal in the cell.
Lordosis	A pronounced concave curve in the back.
Lytic lesions	These refer to abnormalities in the bone that are identified usually by X-rays. Because of bony destruction that occurs in a spotty fashion, the bones look as though holes have been punched out in them — a so-called moth-eaten appearance.
M-band, M-protein Macrophages	Myeloma protein or monoclonal protein. Soft tissue cells that provide a scavenger function
Maintenance therapy	Lower intensity treatment for patients who have achieved a reasonable level of response, e.g. complete response, where the aim of treatment is to maintain this good level of response with the least toxicity.
Malignant	Malicious; cancerous.
Mesenteric vein thrombosis	Blood clots in the intestine's blood vessel system.
Metastasis	Spread of cancer cells.
MGUS	A pre-MM state in which an M-protein is detected but the patient without significant clinical abnormalities that warrant treatment.
Monoclonal	Of a single clone.
Monoclonal antibody	When antibodies (see above) are produced by a single clone of plasma cells, the antibody is called a monoclonal antibody.
Monoclonal protein	Myeloma protein or M-protein.
MRI scan	Investigative body scans that use magnetic waves rather than X-rays for detection.

Multiple myeloma	A cancer of cells of the immune system called plasma cells. Normal plasma cells produce antibodies. Since each plasma cell can only produce one type of antibody, cancerous plasma cells that are all identical (or clonal) all produce only one type of antibody. Thus massive amounts of this single antibody (called the myeloma protein or M-protein) accumulates in multiple myeloma.
Myelin sheathe	This is the insulating layer of nerve tissue that wraps around nerves that prevents cross circuiting and improves electrical conduction.
Myelomagenesis	The biological process that lead to the development of MM.
Nephrotoxicity	Toxicity to kidney function.
Oncogene	Cancer gene.
Oncoprotein	Cancer protein.
Opiate	Substances related to the narcotic drug, opium. e.g. morphine.
Osteoblast	A bone cell that makes bone.
Osteoblastic	Referring to bony abnormalities that have excess bone.
Osteoclast	A bone cell that removes (resorbs) bone.
Osteopenia	Referring to bone thinning.
Osteolytic	Referring to bony abnormalities that totally lack bone.
Pancytopenia	Low blood count involving all 3 major blood cell series — red cells, white cells and platelets.
Parabiosis	An experiment involving two living animals. These animals are usually littermates (siblings) that have the ability to share their blood supplies without adverse effects. If one surgically connects their blood supplies (arteries and veins), blood from one animal can freely enter the other littermate, and vice versa. This is called parabiosis. If there is a condition that is

	present in 1 littermate and not the other, free exchange of blood may reversibly affect the other after parabiosis is performed.
Paraprotein	Another name for monoclonal protein.
Parathyroid	A normal hormonal gland that lies on the sides of the thyroid gland in the neck. It secretes hormones that regulate calcium levels in the body.
Pathological fractures	Usually bones break when a sizable force is applied to them, as when there has been a traumatic accident/injury. When bones fracture after trivial injury, there must be something wrong with the strength of that bone; e.g. a disease or pathology in the bone. Pathological fractures occur at the sites of diseased bone following the slightest of trauma or injury.
Peripheral neuropathy	The nervous system is typically considered to be in two regions — central and peripheral. When the peripheral nerves are affected, e.g. numbness or pins and needles, the nervous condition is known as a peripheral neuropathy.
PET scan	Investigative body scans that use a decaying metabolic tracer that releases positrons rather than X-rays for detection.
Plasma cell	A cell belonging to the immune system that produces antibodies.
Plasma cell leukemia	A very aggressive form of MM in which MM cells are found not only in the bone marrow but also in the peripheral blood.
Plasmablastic MM	A very aggressive form of MM in which MM cells resemble leukemia cells.
Plasmacytoma	Plasma cell tumor.
Polyclonal	Of many clones.
Polyclonal antibody	When antibodies (see above) are produced by many different clones of plasma cells, the antibody is called a polyclonal antibody.

Portal pyemia	Infection of the blood that flows into the liver.
Prednisolone	A glucocorticoid (see above) or steroid drug.
Proto-oncogene	A gene that is presumed to function like a cancer gene.
Proto-oncoprotein	A protein that is presumed to function like a cancer protein.
Radiotherapy	Treatment of cancer using radioactive gamma rays. Like chemotherapy, radiotherapy induces damage to both cancer cells as well as normal cells.
Receptor	A molecule (usually on the surface of the cell) that is used by the cell to communicate with external signals. When engaged, the receptor is able to then produce intracellular signals that produce changes in cellular function.
Renal	Pertaining to the kidneys.
Renal tubules	Small tube-like structures in the kidneys where urine is processed for excretion.
Retinitis	Inflammation (infection) of the retina of the eye.
Risk-adapted therapy	The selection of appropriate therapies based on the perceived prognostic risk of the patient.
Standard deviation	A statistical method of defining the limits of normality.
Standard therapy	In today's context, this usually refers to chemotherapy with or without radiotherapy. Some doctors will include autologous hematopoietic stem cell transplantation as standard therapy but this is not universally practiced.
Stem cells	Cells that are capable of self-division to produce daughter cells. Moreover, these daughter cells are capable of becoming a variety of cell types (i.e. they are not confined to a single cell type).

T cells/ lymphocytes	Cells of the immune system that eventually become killer cells or suppressor cells. T lymphocytes are thought to be the conductors of the immune system.
Targeted Therapies	Treatment that is very precise in targeting specific biological processes that are restricted to cancer cells and not normal cells. The analogy is "smart bombing."
Transformation	In the context of cancer, this means the transition from non-cancer (the benign) to cancer (malignancy).
Translation research	This refers to research that brings products from the research bench to the patient. There are three stages of rigorous testing — (i) in the laboratory (*in vitro* testing), (ii) in research animals (*in vivo* testing), and finally (iii) in humans (clinical trials).
Waldenstrom's macro-globulinemia	A MM-like disorder that is characterized by very high levels of IgM.

LIST OF FIGURES

Figure 2.1	Decision-making Diagnosis-Prognosis Grid	16
Figure 2.2	Simple Risk-adapted Treatment Grid	17
Figure 3.1	The Key to Individualized Therapy for MM	27
Figure 4.1	Four Core Parameters — Triangular Pyramid	33
Figure 4.2	Four Core Parameters — Venn Diagram	33
Figure 4.3	The Triangle in the Corner — "Cure"	41
Figure 4.4	Status of Current Therapies	42
Figure 4.5	Treatment Algorithm for MM in the 1990s and Early 2000s	43
Figure 4.6	Current Status of Conventional Chemotherapy for MM	45
Figure 5.1	Patient Compliance Parameters	50
Figure 5.2	Resources at the Time of Diagnosis	66
Figure 5.3	Depletion of Resources with Fixed Funds During Treatment	67
Figure 5.4	Depletion of Resources Where New Funds are Found During Treatment	68
Figure 5.5	Depletion of Resources Where Unlimited New Funds are Found During Treatment	68

173

Figure 5.6	Impact of Aggressive Therapies on Resources	69
Figure 5.7	Impact of Moderate Therapies on Resources	70
Figure 6.1	MM Parameters	74
Figure 6.2	Basic Concepts of Molecular Interactions	78
Figure 6.3	Hypothetical Examples of the Complexity of Cancer Proteins	79
Figure 6.4	Bare Bones About MM	85
Figure 6.5	MM Clonality	85
Figure 6.6	CD40 and IL-4 Triggering in iCSR	91
Figure 6.7	Co-localization of CD40 and Ku86 on the Cell Membrane of MM Cells	94
Figure 6.8	Ku86v-N — Loss of DNA Repair Function	98
Figure 6.9	Ku86v-C — Putative Oncoprotein	99
Figure 6.10	MM-OC Interaction	107
Figure 6.11	Ultra-high Dose Rate Zoledronic Acid Patient 1	116
Figure 6.12	Ultra-high Dose Rate Zoledronic Acid Patient 2	117
Figure 6.13	Ultra-high Dose Rate Zoledronic Acid Patient 3	119
Figure 6.14	The "Monocyte Loop"	123
Figure 6.15	Monocytosis in MM Patients	124
Figure 6.16	Blockade of the "Monocyte Loop" by Zoledronic acid	125
Figure 6.17	Dose-dependent "Monocyte Loop" Blockade by Zoledronic Acid	126
Figure 6.18	Clinical Outcome After "Monocyte Loop" Blockade by Zoledronic Acid	127
Figure 6.19	High-frequency (3-weekly) Zoledronic Acid — Index Patient	128
Figure 6.20	Critical Level of AMCO Reduction — <200/µL	129
Figure 6.21	Decreased BM Tregs in a Patient Successfully Treated with "dtZ"	136

List of Figures   175

Figure 6.22	Increased BM Tregs in a Patient with Progressive Disease After "dtZ"	137
Figure 6.23	Percentage of BM Tregs Correlates with Depth of Response in Patients Treated with "dtZ"	137
Figure 7.1	Current Treatment Parameters	141
Figure 7.2	The "dtZ" Regimen	143
Figure 7.3	The "dtZ" Regimen — Relapsed/ Refractory Patients	146
Figure 7.4	The "dtZ" Regimen — New Patients	147
Figure 8.1	Future Opportunities Parameters	151

LIST OF TABLES

Table 2.1	Experience, Experiment, Evidence and Execution	10
Table 2.2A	The Basis for a Diagnostic Grid Based on Whether to Treat	12
Table 2.2B	"Treat" or "Don't Treat" Grid	12
Table 2.3	A Proposed Improvement of the Diagnostic-Treatment Grid	14
Table 2.4	Summary of the ISS Staging System	15
Table 3.1	Concluding Clinical Trial Findings	21
Table 4.1	Group Dynamics Analysis of MM Treatment Strategies	40
Table 4.2	Here Lies the Future	46
Table 5.1	The Basis of Immunoprotective Agents in MM	59
Table 6.1	CD40L and/or IL-4 Triggering of MM Cells and Normal B Cells and Cell Proliferation	92
Table 6.2	CD40L and/or IL-4 Triggering of MM Cells and Normal B Cells and CD40-Ku86 Co-localization	95
Table 6.3	Characteristics of Ku86 Variants in MM Cells	96
Table 6.4	Zoledronic Acid's Effects in the SCID-hu Mouse Model of MM	108

Table 6.5	Use of Zoledronic Acid in Human Clinical Trials — Dose Considerations	110
Table 6.6	Use of Zoledronic Acid in Human Clinical Trials — Efficacy	111
Table 6.7	Dose Equivalence (EQmg) of Zoledronic Acid	113
Table 6.8	Dose equivalence (EQmg) of 3-weekly and Monthly Zoledronic Acid	114
Table 6.9	Effect of Body Size on Dosing Rate of Zoledronic Acid	114
Table 6.10	Ultra-high Dose Rate of Zoledronic Acid	115
Table 6.11	Simple Immunology	131
Table 6.12	Some Markers of Immunodeficiency in MM	132
Table 6.13	The Concept of "Stage Zero"	138

REFERENCES

1. Durie BG, Salmon SE. (1975) A clinical staging system for multiple myeloma. Correlation of measured myeloma cell mass with presenting clinical features, response to treatment, and survival. *Cancer* **36**(3):842–54.
2. Kyle RA, *et al.* (2003) Criteria for the classification of monoclonal gammopathies, multiple myeloma and related disorders: a report of the International Myeloma Working Group. *Br J Haematol* **121**(5): 749–57.
3. http://myeloma.org/main.jsp?type=article&id=1045
4. http://www.multiplemyeloma.org/about_myeloma/2.05.php
5. Agnelli L, Bicciato S, Mattioli M, *et al.* (2005) Molecular classification of multiple myeloma: a distinct transcriptional profile characterizes patients expressing CCND1 and negative for 14q32 translocations. *J Clin Oncol* **23**(29):7296–306.
6. Zhan F, Huang Y, Colla S, *et al.* (2006) The molecular classification of multiple myeloma. *Blood* **108**(6):2020–8.
7. Greipp PR, San Miguel J, Durie BG, *et al.* (2005) International staging system for multiple myeloma. *J Clin Oncol* **23**(15):3412–20.
8. Tan D, Hwang W, Koh LP, Teoh G. (2005) High response and complete remission rates in Asian patients with relapsed/refractory multiple myeloma treated with bortezomib. *Proc 10th Eur Haematol Assoc Congress 2005,* abstr 0925.
9. Teoh G, Tan D, Hwang W, *et al.* (2005) High response and complete remission rates in relapsed/refractory multiple myeloma treated with

bortezomib, thalidomide, dexamethasone and zoledronic acid (VTD-Z) combination therapy. *Blood* **106**(11):abstr 5127.

10. Teoh G, Tan D, Hwang W, *et al.* (2006) Addition of bortezomib to thalidomide, dexamethasone and zoledronic acid (VTD-Z regimen) significantly improves complete remission rates in patients with relapsed/refractory multiple myeloma. *J Clin Oncol* **18S**(I):683s; abstr 17537.

11. Durie BG, Harousseau JL, Miguel JS, *et al.* (2006) International Myeloma Working Group. International uniform response criteria for multiple myeloma. *Leukemia* **20**(9):1467–73.

12. Urashima M, Ogata A, Chauhan D, *et al.* (1996) Interleukin-6 promotes multiple myeloma cell growth via phosphorylation of retinoblastoma protein. *Blood* **88**(6):2219–27.

13. Chauhan D, Kharbanda S, Ogata A, *et al.* (1997) Interleukin-6 inhibits Fas-induced apoptosis and stress-activated protein kinase activation in multiple myeloma cells. *Blood* **89**(1):227–34.

14. Urashima M, Teoh G, Chauhan D, *et al.* (1997) Interleukin-6 overcomes p21WAF1 upregulation and G1 growth arrest induced by dexamethasone and interferon-gamma in multiple myeloma cells. *Blood* **90**(1):279–89.

15. Ogata A, Chauhan D, Teoh G, *et al.* (1997) IL-6 triggers cell growth via the Ras-dependent mitogen-activated protein kinase cascade. *J Immunol* **159**(5):2212–21.

16. http://www.nccn.org/

17. Teoh G, Tan D, Hwang W, *et al.* (2006) Use of immunoglobulin infusions in the management of bortezomib-induced peripheral neuropathy in multiple myeloma. *Blood* **108**(11) (Suppl):363b; abstr 5097.

18. Manochakian R, Miller KC, Chanan-Khan AA. (2007) Clinical impact of bortezomib in frontline regimens for patients with multiple myeloma. *Oncologist* **12**:978–90.

19. Chauhan D, Pandey P, Ogata A, *et al.* (1997) Cytochrome c-dependent and -independent induction of apoptosis in multiple myeloma cells. *J Biol Chem* **272**(48):29995–7.

20. Teoh G, Anderson KC. (1997) Interaction of tumor and host cells with adhesion and extracellular matrix molecules in the

development of multiple myeloma. *Hematol Oncol Clin North Am* **11**(1):27–42.

21. Bergsagel PL, Nardini E, Brents L, Chesi M, Kuehl WM. (1997) IgH translocations in multiple myeloma: a nearly universal event that rarely involves c-myc. *Curr Top Microbiol Immunol* **224**:283–7.

22. Teoh G, Tai YT, Urashima M, *et al.* (2000) CD40 activation mediates p53-dependent cell cycle regulation in human multiple myeloma cell lines. *Blood* **95**(3):1039–46.

23. Teoh G, Urashima M, Greenfield EA, *et al.* (1998) The 86-kD subunit of Ku autoantigen mediates homotypic and heterotypic adhesion of multiple myeloma cells. *J Clin Invest* **101**(6):1379–88.

24. Morio T, Hanissian SH, Bacharier LB, *et al.* (1999) Ku in the cytoplasm associates with CD40 in human B cells and translocates into the nucleus following incubation with IL-4 and anti-CD40 mAb. *Immunity* **11**(3):339–48.

25. Tai YT, Teoh G, Lin B, *et al.* (2000) Ku86 variant expression and function in multiple myeloma cells is associated with increased sensitivity to DNA damage. *J Immunol* **165**(11):6347–55.

26. Gullo C, Au M, Feng G, Teoh G. (2006) The biology of Ku and its potential oncogenic role in cancer. *Biochim Biophys Acta* **1765**(2):223–34.

27. Gullo CA, Ge F, Cow G, Teoh G. (2008) Ku86 exists as both a full-length and a protease-sensitive natural variant in multiple myeloma cells. *Cancer Cell Int* **8**:4.

28. Hwang WYK, Gullo CA, Shen J, *et al.* Decoupling of normal CD40/interleukin-4 immunoglobulin heavy chain switch signal leads to genomic instability in RPMI 8226 and SGH-MM5 multiple myeloma cell lines. *Leukemia* **20**(4):715–23.

29. Teoh G, Anderson KC. (1999) The culture, characterization, and triggering of B lymphocytes. In: Koller MR and Palsson BO (eds.), Human Cell Culture, Vol. IV: *Primary Hematopoietic Cells*, Kluwer Academic Publishers, The Netherlands, pp. 101–24.

30. Bataille R, Chappard D, Marcelli C, *et al.* Recruitment of new osteoblasts and osteoclasts is the earliest critical event in the pathogenesis of human multiple myeloma. *J Clin Invest* **88**:62–6.

31. Roodman GD. (1995) Osteoclast function in Paget's disease and multiple myeloma. *Bone* **17**:57S-61S.
32. Roodman GD. (2004) Pathogenesis of myeloma bone disease. *Blood Cells Mol Dis* **32**:290–2.
33. Urashima M, Chen BP, Chen S, *et al.* (1997) The development of a model for the homing of multiple myeloma cells to human bone marrow. *Blood* **90**:754–65.
34. Zangari M, Esseltine D, Lee CK, *et al.* (2005) Response to bortezomib is associated to osteoblastic activation in patients with multiple myeloma. *Br J Haematol* **131**:71–3.
35. Caligaris-Cappio F, Gregoretti MG, Ghia P, Bergui L. (1992) In vitro growth of human multiple myeloma: implications for biology and therapy. *Hematol Oncol Clin North Am* **6**:257–71.
36. Caligaris-Cappio F, Gregoretti MG, Merico F, *et al.* (1992) Bone marrow microenvironment and the progression of multiple myeloma. *Leuk Lymphoma* **8**:15–22.
37. Yaccoby S, Pearse RN, Johnson CL, *et al.* (2002) Myeloma interacts with the bone marrow microenvironment to induce osteoclastogenesis and is dependent on osteoclast activity. *Br J Haematol* **116**:278–90.
38. Rosen LS, Gordon D, Kaminski M, *et al.* (2001) Zoledronic acid versus pamidronate in the treatment of skeletal metastases in patients with breast cancer or osteolytic lesions of multiple myeloma: a phase III, double-blind, comparative trial. *Cancer J* **7**:377–87.
39. Rosen LS, Gordon D, Tchekmedyian NS, *et al.* (2004) Long-term efficacy and safety of zoledronic acid in the treatment of skeletal metastases in patients with nonsmall cell lung carcinoma and other solid tumors: a randomized, Phase III, double-blind, placebo-controlled trial. *Cancer* **100**:2613–21.
40. Mundy GR, Yoneda T, Hiraga T. (2001) Preclinical studies with zoledronic acid and other bisphosphonates: impact on the bone microenvironment. *Semin Oncol* **28**:35–44.
41. Croucher P, Jagdev S, Coleman R. (2003) The anti-tumor potential of zoledronic acid. *Breast* **12** (Suppl 2):S30–36.
42. Rosen LS, Gordon D, Kaminski M, *et al.* (2003) Long-term efficacy and safety of zoledronic acid compared with pamidronate disodium in

the treatment of skeletal complications in patients with advanced multiple myeloma or breast carcinoma: a randomized, double-blind, multicenter, comparative trial. *Cancer* **98**:1735–44.

43. Bataille R, Magub M, Grenier J, *et al.* (1982) Serum beta-2-microglobulin in multiple myeloma: relation to presenting features and clinical status. *Eur J Cancer Clin Oncol* **18**:59–66.

44. Bataille R, Grenier J, Sany J. (1984) Beta-2-microglobulin in myeloma: optimal use for staging, prognosis, and treatment — a prospective study of 160 patients. *Blood* **63**:468–76.

45. Durie BG, Katz M, Crowley J. (2005) Osteonecrosis of the jaw and bisphosphonates. *N Engl J Med* **353**:99–102; discussion 199–102.

46. Maerevoet M, Martin C, Duck L. (2005) Osteonecrosis of the jaw and bisphosphonates. *N Engl J Med* **353**:99–102; discussion 199–102.

47. Bamias A, Kastritis E, Bamia C, *et al.* (2005) Osteonecrosis of the jaw in cancer after treatment with bisphosphonates: incidence and risk factors. *J Clin Oncol* **23**:8580–7.

48. Durie BG, Katz M, Crowley J. (2005) Osteonecrosis of the jaw and bisphosphonates. *N Engl J Med* **353**:99–102; discussion 199–102.

49. Maerevoet M, Martin C, Duck L. (2005) Osteonecrosis of the jaw and bisphosphonates. *N Engl J Med* **353**:99–102; discussion 199–102.

50. Bamias A, Kastritis E, Bamia C, *et al.* (2005) Osteonecrosis of the jaw in cancer after treatment with bisphosphonates: incidence and risk factors. *J Clin Oncol* **23**:8580–7.

51. Richardson PG, Barlogie B, Berenson J, *et al.* (2005) Clinical factors predictive of outcome with bortezomib in patients with relapsed, refractory multiple myeloma. *Blood* **106**:2977–81.

52. Walker DG. (1973) Osteopetrosis cured by temporary parabiosis. *Science* **180**:875.

53. Massey HM, Flanagan AM. (1999) Human osteoclasts derive from CD14-positive monocytes. *Br J Haematol* **106**:167–70.

54. Nicholson GC, Malakellis M, Collier FM, *et al.* (2000) Induction of osteoclasts from CD14-positive human peripheral blood mononuclear cells by receptor activator of nuclear factor kappaB ligand (RANKL). *Clin Sci (Lond)* **99**:133–40.

55. Roodman GD. (2002) Role of the bone marrow microenvironment in multiple myeloma. *J Bone Miner Res* **17**:1921–5.

56. Sewell RL. (1977) Lymphocyte abnormalities in myeloma. *Br J Haematol* **36**:545–51.
57. Kraj M, Krzeminska-Lawkowiczowa I, Lawkowicz W, *et al.* (1979) Lysozyme in the serum, urine and peripheral blood leukocytes in patients with immunocytoma. *Arch Immunol Ther Exp (Warsz)* **27**:875–88.
58. Blom J, Nielsen H, Larsen SO, Mansa B. (1984) A study of certain functional parameters of monocytes from patients with multiple myeloma: comparison with monocytes from healthy individuals. *Scand J Haematol* **33**:425–31.
59. Natazuka T, Yamaguchi T, Murayama T, *et al.* (1994) Chronic myelomonocytic leukemia following prolonged alkylating agent therapy for multiple myeloma. *Int J Hematol* **60**:263–5.
60. Matano S, Nakamura S, Kobayashi K, *et al.* (1996) Acute myelomono-cytic leukaemia with 11q23 abnormality during multiple myeloma: is this related to anthracycline? *Acta Haematol* **95**:144–7.
61. Yoshida K, Aida K, Horibe T, *et al.* (1997) Plasma cell leukemia asso-ciated with monocytosis. *Rinsho Ketsueki* **38**:604–9.
62. Galasko CS. (1982) Mechanisms of lytic and blastic metastatic disease of bone. *Clin Orthop Relat Res* **169**:20–7.
63. Berenson JR. (2001) New advances in the biology and treatment of myeloma bone disease. *Semin Hematol* **38**:15–20.
64. Green JR. (2002) Chemical and biological prerequisites for novel bisphosphonate molecules: results of comparative preclinical studies. *Semin Oncol* **28**:4–10.
65. Brown RD, Pope B, Yuen E, *et al.* (1998) The expression of T cell related costimulatory molecules in multiple myeloma. *Leuk Lymphoma* **31**:379–84.
66. Teoh G, Tan D, Hwang W, *et al.* (2006) Factors influencing responsiveness to bortezomib in patients with multiple myeloma suggest a possible role for host immunocompetency. *Blood* **108**(11) (Suppl):364b; abstr 5100.
67. Koh LP, Hwang W, Ng HJ, *et al.* (2002) Higher doses of zoledronic acid induce in vivo anti-osteoclast as well as anti-tumor effects in patients with multiple myeloma. *Blood* **100**(11) (Suppl):391b; abstr 5126.

68. Teoh G, Hwang W, Koh LP, *et al.* (2004) Low dose dexamethasone and thalidomide with higher frequency zoledronic acid (dtZ) for multiple myeloma. *Blood* **104**(11): abstr 4915.
69. Teoh G, Hwang W, Koh LP, *et al.* (2005) Low dose dexamethasone and thalidomide with higher frequency zoledronic acid (dtZ) for relapsed/refractory multiple myeloma. *Haematologica* **90** (Suppl 1):141–2; abstr PO.710.
70. Teoh G, Hwang W, Koh LP, *et al.* (2007) The "dtZ" palliative regimen for relapsed/ refractory MM. *Haematologica* **92** (Suppl 2):170; abstr PO655.

INDEX

Autologous hemopoietic stem
cell transplantation, 44

Blood supply, 73, 76, 82, 121,
123, 129
Bone marrow microenvironment,
34, 102
Bone remodeling, 104

Cancer cell lines, 36, 102
CD40, 40, 90, 91, 94–96, 98,
100, 101
Clinical trials, 20–22, 27, 141,
148
Clonality, 82, 85, 86
Compliance, 29, 31, 49, 50

Drug discovery, 107–121, 154,
155

Evidence-based medicine, 9,
10, 140, 147

Family and friends, 49, 57

Gene expression profiling, 9, 84
Genetic signatures, 12, 16, 133
Group dynamics, 26, 27, 76,
140, 141
Growth factors, 81, 106, 122,
123, 132

Immune system, 73, 76, 82, 88,
130, 131, 134, 135, 138
Immunoglobulin isotype
class switch recombination,
86
Infections, 58–60, 69
Investigator-initiated trials, 48,
154

Ku86, 88, 89, 93–97, 100

Monocyte loop, 122,
123, 125–127, 129,
130
Motivation, 29, 31, 32, 54,
60–63, 71
Mouse models, 106, 108

187

Multiple myeloma, bone
disease, 2, 3, 6, 103, 105,
107, 111, 112, 124
Multiple myeloma, clinical
presentation, 2–7, 51–54
Multiple myeloma, diagnosis, 8,
12
Multiple myeloma, disease
biology, 72, 73
Myelomagenesis, 87, 88

Oncoproteins, 83–86, 95, 99
Optimal therapy, 17, 18,
142–145
Osteoblasts, 104
Osteoclasts, 104, 107

Parabiosis, 121, 122

Regulating healthcare, 150,
156
Regulatory T lymphocytes, 130
Resources, 49, 54, 57, 63–71
Risk-adapted therapy, 17

Sponsors, academic, 150, 151,
154
Sponsors, investors, 150, 155
Sponsors, pharmaceutical
companies, 150, 154

Tolerance and will power, 60,
61
Treatment, chemotherapy,
41–45
Treatment, choices, 17, 43
Treatment, maintenance
therapy, 139
Treatment, response, 24
Treatment, targeted therapies,
35
Treatment, weaning off therapy,
138

Zoledronic acid, equivalent
dose (EQmg), 112, 113,
115
Zoledronic acid, ultra-high
dose, 114–121, 129, 130